THE COITUS CHRONICLES

THE COITUS CHRONICLES

My Quest for Sex, Love, and Orgasms

OLIVE PERSIMMON

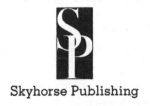

Skyhorse Publishing

Skyhorse Publishing books may be purchased in bulk at special discounts for sales promotion, corporate gifts, fund-raising, or educational purposes. Special editions can also be created to specifications. For details, contact the Special Sales Department, Skyhorse Publishing, 307 West 36th Street, 11th Floor, New York, NY 10018 or info@skyhorsepublishing.com.

Skyhorse® and Skyhorse Publishing® are registered trademarks of Skyhorse Publishing, Inc.®, a Delaware corporation.

Visit our website at www.skyhorsepublishing.com.

10 9 8 7 6 5 4 3 2 1

Library of Congress Cataloging-in-Publication Data is available on file.

Cover design by Erin Seaward-Hiatt

Print ISBN: 978-1-5107-3241-4
Ebook ISBN: 978-1-5107-3244-5

Printed in the United States of America

coitus

noun co·i·tus \ ˈkō-ə-təs, kō-ˈē-, ˈkȯi-təs \

Physical union of male and female genitalia accompanied
by rhythmic movements.*

Also, a fancy way of saying sex.

Anyone who uses it is probably not having sex.

---

* As copied and pasted from www.merriam-webster.com.

CONTENTS

When I started this book, sex, for me, meant a penis entering my vagina. I'll be the first one to acknowledge that my scope was limited and naive. Thankfully I learned that sex means a whole lot more than that to a whole lot of people.

This book is for anyone who feels as insecure and confused as I did about sex. It's for anyone who thinks that everyone else is having more, better, and kinkier sex than them.

WE'RE IN THIS TOGETHER.

THE COITUS
CHRONICLES

THE BRIEF HISTORY OF AN UNINTENTIONAL CELIBATE

There are a few things you need to know about me before reading this book.

1. I'm twenty-nine and the last time I had sex was four years, five months, three days, and 1.3 hours ago.
2. I've had intercourse with two people, less than eleven times in total.
3. I've never done reverse cowgirl.

Or doggy-style.

Or anything with whipped cream.

I wrote a book about my tenantless vagina called *Unintentionally Celibate* and my love life has only gone downhill from there.

Maybe you've already pegged me as some sort of undateable weirdo who smells like onions. Let me assure you, and you'll have to take my word for it, I don't smell like onions. And although I don't look like Angelina Jolie I can more or less hold my own at a bar.

So how did I wind up here?

Here being a desolate wasteland of no sex. A Sexmageddon. A Coitus Catastrophe.

It's a question I've asked myself ad nauseam for the past four years, five months, three days, and 1.3 hours.

My friends are surprised that I'm in this sexless situation.

Honestly, I'm not. I kind of saw this coming.

It hasn't been smooth sailing for me in the romance department. As far back as middle school, when other girls were discovering their feminine charms, not one single boy at Klimpton D. Walton Intermediate School "like liked" me.

Not one.

Granted, I did look exactly like Danny DeVito.

I was seriously overweight with nerdy glasses. My mom bought all my clothes, which meant that I was wearing pom-pom glitter sweatshirts well into seventh grade. My hobbies included volunteering at the nursing home across the street, crafting, theater, and sitting in the middle of my front yard in my inflatable chair.

Needless to say, I wasn't killing it in the middle school dating scene.

In high school, when other people started exploring sex, I still said "fiddlesticks" instead of "fuck," and boys were uncharted territory.

When it came to sex, everything I knew I learned by cybering and downloading illegal porn on Napster.

Which means I knew NOTHING about sex.

To this day, my knowledge of the female anatomy is often ill-informed. Case in point: I thought it was possible to lose a NuvaRing inside of you until a friend of mine informed me that my vagina "wasn't the gateway to Narnia" and things couldn't get lost in it.*

---

* The NuvaRing is a type of birth control. It's a magic rubber band coated with hormones that you stick in your vagina and somehow it stops you from having babies.

I blamed my midwestern education for my lack of knowledge, but none of my friends had this problem. Perhaps I just wasn't paying attention during sex ed because sex wasn't even on my mind.

I didn't talk to boys until I was fifteen.

My first kiss? Sixteen.

My first kiss without a face full of slobber? Eighteen.

At twenty-four, I lost my virginity to a Ken doll look-alike who cared less about me than I'd like to admit. We had sex a total of eight times and never moved beyond missionary. We broke up after I came over to his house without any underwear on and he decided to build his patio table instead of sleeping with me.

Not the best introduction into the world of sex.

My next partner was my long-term friend with benefits, Tyler. On and off for two years, we exchanged oral pleasantries, but surprisingly, never had penetrative sex.

Until one night we did. Three times. He was a gentle, giving lover. He kissed parts of my body that Ken doll had ignored. We went to the grocery store afterward and held hands.

It was Sexual Redemption.

It was also the last time I had sex.

I moved to the Big Apple one month later.

There's a rite of passage when you move to NYC that involves owning no furniture, having no friends, and sobbing on the subway once a week. No job, no money, and as a result, no self-esteem. Dating was off the table.

It wasn't until I was finally settled that I felt good enough about myself to start dating again. There were first dates. Second dates that never turned into third dates. Some make out sessions. Some over-the-pants penis touching. Under-the-pants scrotum stroking. Sexual innuendos. Occasional nipple-licking, butt-grabbing, thigh-stroking nights full of potential.

But no sex.

A few years into the dry spell, I started dating someone seriously but *still* didn't have sex with him. By then it had become a thing. I was afraid that because I was inexperienced, I'd be bad in bed. In my mind, that was practically the most embarrassing thing a person could be. I had so many insecurities that I kept putting off sex until our relationship ended before we could do the no-pants penetration dance.

Luckily, everything changed on a Sunday night in November. By a twist of fate, I wound up at a party with a select group of members from one of New York's sex-positive communities.

I had no idea what "sex-positive" even meant.

I had been invited to the party by my friend Renee, who, unbeknownst to me, was an active participant in the community. According to her, the sex-positive community was based on the belief that sex was natural and healthy, that it should be enjoyed. She and her friends talked openly about intercourse, went to sexy parties, and occasionally participated in polyamorous relationships. They enthusiastically explored new ways to seek pleasure.

I was oblivious to all of this until I walked in on the middle of a conversation about OM'ing. The only time I'd ever heard the word "om" was in relation to yoga. I was on a yoga kick so I joined in eagerly ready to discuss Downward-Facing Dog.

When someone mentioned their clitoris, I knew we weren't talking about any form of yoga I was familiar with. Seeing the confusion on my face, Renee told me about Orgasmic Meditation, or OM'ing for short, a meditative technique where one person stroked another person's clitoris during a timed session.

I stared at her blankly in response.

Renee said, "I could explain it to you, but it might be better for you to just try it. Maybe this is what you need to unblock your own sexual energy because clearly something's amiss."

I wanted to deny this but she was right. My mojo was broken and I had no idea how to fix it.

"This is your next book," Renee said. "You should spend a year exploring a sex-positive lifestyle in NYC."

I began to protest. "I don't like cas—"

"Casual sex," Renee said. "Yeah, I know. Everyone knows. That's not what I'm suggesting. I'm saying that you should be more open to learning about what's out there. You don't remotely try when it comes to your love life."

I folded my arms across my chest defensively.

"I try. I'm just . . . busy," I said.

"Okay, sure, but let's say you were open to it, there's a ton of things you could explore," she said.

Everyone in the circle brainstormed sexy adventures for me. As they threw out ideas, I remained silent, thinking about the proposition: Explore sex and dating. Fix my love life. Write about it.

It sounded like a terrible idea. My parents would be embarrassed. My employer would fire me. Strangers on the Internet would troll me.

As I continued to come up with reasons to say "no," a small voice was telling me that instead of ruining my life, it just might save me. For four years I had been doing things a certain way and it wasn't working. I *had* to do something differently. If I didn't, I was going to die alone with a tombstone that read:

Here lies Olive. She never tried reverse cowgirl.

"I can't believe I'm saying this . . . but maybe."

Renee squealed with excitement.

"My friend Sheng is a sex guru and OM'ing coach. You should connect with him, he might have ideas," she said.

I left the party feeling excited and scared; it was fun to talk about, but I probably wasn't going to go through with any of it.

The next morning Renee unintentionally forced my hand by sending an email introducing me to Sheng telling him that I was exploring the sex-positive lifestyle. She made me seem like an adventurous badass, ready and willing to try everything, which was laughably far from the truth.

"How exciting," Sheng wrote in his email back. "My friend is hosting a BDSM class this Saturday. He's one of the best instructors in the city. If you want to come, I can get you a free ticket."

I didn't respond for three days. Replying to his email meant that I was doing this. That I was accepting the challenge to confront my own discomfort with sexuality and my non-existent love life.

I wanted to call it off. I wanted to go back to bed, binge-watch *Gilmore Girls*, and forget I ever received any email at all.

Yet, that was the exact same fear that got me into this situation in the first place.

Which is why I wrote: "I'll see you Saturday."

Just like that, the Coitus Chronicles began. . . .

KNOT WHAT YOU THINK

It was the day before class and I was freaking out. Not only was I terrified about going to a BDSM lesson, I had no idea what to wear. I imagined whips and handcuffs over my tan cowl-neck sweater.

I pulled out my leather pants and a black top and called Renee.

"No, no," she said. "Don't wear leather or too much black; that screams newbie. Don't wear a tight necklace either; that means you're collared."

I had no idea what that meant, which made it glaringly obvious that I was in over my head. My only experience with BDSM was from reading *Fifty Shades of Grey*, which obviously wasn't the handbook for an intro to kink.

I'd only ever had vanilla sex.

Boring, missionary sex. Kind-of-sweaty-but-not-*THAT*-sweaty sex.

I hadn't even done shower stuff. It was all uncharted territory.

Yet here I was, registered for a BDSM class. It was like learning to drive before learning to walk. I still needed my nooky training wheels for God's sake.

On the day of, I took the train down to Brooklyn. I was expecting a dimly lit dungeon, so I was surprised when I walked into a multi-purpose yoga studio that smelled like peppermint. It was light and airy, with rows of folding chairs facing a man sitting on a stool. There were no visible signs that this was a BDSM class. Our instructor's name was Mr. Rao and he was . . . normal-looking; no eyeliner or studded chokers.

All the seats were taken except for the one directly in front of our instructor in the first row. I sat down, waiting anxiously for class to begin.

Mr. Rao looked around the room, smiling at his students before saying, "BDSM stands for bondage, dominance and submission, and sadomasochism. Today, we're going to focus on the first three. Are you ready to play?"

I looked around the room too. There were fifteen people in class including myself.

My eyes landed on the woman next to me. She was wearing a see-through shirt.

Her stomach growled loudly.

"Sorry, honey. My IBS kicks in sometimes," she whispered, pulling out a comically large container of Metamucil. I smiled back at her.

"I want to find out *why* you're here. A lot of this class is going to be us talking," Rao said. Talking I could do. Talking was cool. Usually you couldn't get me to shut up.

He started with an older man in the last row, bald with intense blue eyes.

"When I fuck someone, I want to ravage them. I want to rip them to shreds and use their body for my own pleasure," the man said.

I raised my eyebrows in concern; holy shit, what had I gotten myself into?

The next few answers were milder before Rao finally got to me. He glanced at my name tag and said, "Olive, what brings you here today?"

It was a simple question without a simple answer.

"Um. Well. I haven't had sex in a long time, so I'm trying to do things differently this year," I said.

"How long?"

"About five years."

There was a collective gasp around the room. I was used to that response when people heard the number. You'd have thought I said I was an alien and then pulled off my face to prove it, *Men in Black* style.

"Why not?"

He was pushing me to be honest. It seemed like he pushed everyone to say three more things than they actually wanted to as a way of getting to the truth.

"I . . . uhh . . . want to be in control when it comes to sex," I said, my mouth getting dry.

"There are plenty of men in this room who would love that. Raise your hand if you want her to be in control of you."

Five guys raised their hands. My face turned red as I laughed awkwardly, avoiding their gazes.

"Why is that a problem?" he asked.

"Sometimes I need to be too in control. Like, I make rules and sometimes . . . I'm afraid to be out of control."

"Oh, I see. You make laws about sex. If someone doesn't do and say all the right things, or follow the rules that you've made up, you won't sleep with them."

"Yeah. Something like that," I said.

"That's going to hurt you," he said.

"I know. That's why I'm here. I'm trying to do things differently."

To my immense relief, Rao moved on to someone else. While another woman talked about how she wanted to be tied up, I thought about my need for control. It didn't make sense. I was a big risk-taker in many ways. My life was full of impulsive and adventurous decisions. I moved to NYC without a job, circled the globe without money, posted vulnerable articles on the Internet. But when it came to sex, I was cautious to a fault.

A handsome Irishman caught my attention when he said, "I feel like I'm so far behind everyone else. When it comes to sex and relationships, I'm like a high schooler, scared of talking to girls."

Ah, yes, another member of my tribe. A tribe that no one wanted to belong to: The Sexually Inexperienced. I made a mental note to talk to him later.

The final person to speak was a shy girl named Cody. She told a story about how she'd fooled around with someone because, even though she hadn't really wanted to hook up, she hadn't wanted to hurt his feelings.

Rao looked at her and firmly but compassionately said, "You should have said something and stopped. You should never do anything you don't want to do. It's not your job to support someone else's ego at your own expense. From now on you say something."

Rao stood up, taking in the room, sighing deeply before saying, "There seems to be a common theme here—of guilt. For our first exercise, you're going to confess everything you're ashamed of."

I looked around the room, confused. I didn't understand what that had to do with BDSM.

"Find a partner. One of you will speak and one will listen. The listener will put their fingers in their ears so they can't actually hear. For the speaker, it's about saying it out loud. Maintain eye contact the entire time. Listeners, keep your faces neutral. Give them space. Allow them to be vulnerable."

This was both better and worse than what I had expected. I was fully clothed and there was no whipping, so that was good.

I partnered up with the man who wanted to "ravage women."

I stood across from him and placed my fingers in my ears, making direct eye contact. Despite my best efforts, I could hear everything he was saying. I tried hard not to listen though, because what he was saying scared me.

"I pretend to be a nice guy, but I'm not. It's a lie. I don't care about anyone's pleasure but my own and I want to rage-fuck women. In fact, I want to fuck *you*. I want to fuck you and use you and abuse you."

He smiled maniacally.

Keep your face neutral, I thought. *You're not supposed to be hearing this. This is a safe space to admit any desires. Stay calm.*

It was hard because I was terrified. It was the longest two minutes of my life.

Finally, the time was up and I was grateful. I didn't want to be near him any longer. Even though I was supposed to be non-judgmental, I made a mental note to avoid him for the rest of class; something was off about that guy.

My next partner was an attractive, dark-skinned man in his mid-twenties. His face was angelic, which made him look sweet and kind. He seemed like someone I'd hang out/make out with. I placed my fingers in my ears even though I knew it was a farce and I could hear him anyway.

He looked me directly in the eyes and I felt a connection that I hadn't felt with my last partner.

"I'm ashamed of the color of my skin," he said.

I could feel my heart break, saddened that was the first thing he said.

"I feel ashamed that I'm here today. That I like this stuff. I feel like I'm letting my family down. I'm ashamed that I'm not making more money. I'm ashamed that I'm not further along in my career and I don't know if my life is ever going to come together," he said.

There was nothing psychotic or scary about his gaze. He was just a man, standing before me, vulnerable and human.

More than anything, I felt deep compassion and love for this person.

I wanted to brush my fingers gently across his cheek and say, "Your skin is beautiful and so are you. It's okay that you're here; you're not hurting anyone. We *all* feel like we should be further along." I wanted to caress his face with kisses and whisper in his ear that everything was going to be fine.

But I didn't. Because I wasn't supposed to hear any of it.

So I just kept my face blank and moved on.

Next it was time for the listeners to become the confessors.

I partnered with an older, petite woman with brown eyes. She had offered me some almonds earlier. Her hair was pulled neatly back in a bun.

I stared into the eyes of a woman I had just met and sucked in my breath. She smiled at me. The wrinkles around her eyes indicated that this was a familiar face for her to make. Her sweet-tempered demeanor should have made it easier.

It didn't.

I opened my mouth to speak but the words got stuck.

They had been buried for too long.

I knew she was going to hear everything. Even with her fingers in her ears, she would hear.

"I feel ashamed of . . ." I stumbled over my words and stopped.

It was too hard.

"It's okay," she said, nodding with reassurance.

Tears began to pool in my eyes until finally I said, "I'm embarrassed that I haven't had sex in forever. That I haven't had a lot of sex and I might be bad at it. I feel ashamed that I'm a compulsive overeater . . . that sometimes I treat my body like shit. I feel ashamed that I had to borrow money from a friend to pay my rent, that I'm twenty-nine and still struggling with my finances."

Then for the next two minutes, I told a perfect stranger everything I felt ashamed of.

I told her things I thought I had long forgotten, things that had happened years before, like an STD scare in college and something mean I had said to my first love when I was eighteen.

Another tear rolled down my face. It was one of the hardest things I'd ever done. I felt exposed and self-conscious, but also lighter. There was a weird power in saying things aloud. In some ways, I felt like it freed me from some of that shit I had been carrying around for a long time.

My partner, with her kind eyes, reached out and hugged me, holding me gently as I tried to sniffle discretely.

"Have you made that shame your story?" Rao asked as we found a new partner.

I had. Especially about sex. I was the girl who didn't have sex. It had become ingrained in the narrative I was telling about myself, to myself.

We did it again with our new partners before rejoining the group to sit down. It wasn't any easier the second time around. I cried twice as hard.

I slumped in my seat, hiding my face and my runny mascara. I pulled a tissue out of my purse, and avoided talking or looking at anyone else. I felt gutted and I wanted to be alone.

"And *that* is exactly what BDSM is," Rao said, trying to regain control of the somber energy in the room.

"Being the Dom," he continued, "is about creating space for someone to be *that* level of vulnerable. It's about being 200 percent responsible for that person, making them feel safe enough to trust you with their body. Being a Sub is about being *that* trusting. It's beautiful, isn't it?"

It actually was.

My mind was blown. I had always assumed BDSM was about taking power. I had never dreamed it was also about vulnerability and trust. It challenged everything I thought I knew about BDSM.

"Alright, we're gonna break for lunch, but when we get back we're going to do rope-play," Rao said.

I was still recovering from the exercise and in the middle of a heart-wrenching, life-changing, mascara-dripping-down-my-face moment, when Rao's like, "Okay people, let's get sandwiches."

I stood up to leave even though I wasn't ready for chicken salad and chips.

I walked to a deli and the man at the counter asked me if I was okay. I knew my eyes must have still been red and blotchy. It required too much explaining to say, "Not really, I just confessed all my shame to strangers at a BDSM class." So instead I said, "I'm good. Turkey with mayo on the side please and coffee to go."

I sat on a bench in downtown Brooklyn, picking at my sandwich, feeling emotional and raw until it was time to head back in. I stopped in the bathroom to fix my mascara.

Post-lunch it was rope time.

Instructor Rao pulled out fifteen red, braided ropes. We were going to use the ropes to practice dominance and submission.

He did a demo, folding the top in half and looping the two sides into a knot. We practiced tying the knot a few times to ensure that we got it.

Easy as pie; anyone could tie a freaking knot.

"Now find a partner," Rao said.

Not so simple.

The closest man to me was the one who wanted to fuck me. I didn't want to work with him so I jumped from my seat as quickly as I could and headed toward the cute, inexperienced Irishman.

He was quiet. His demeanor seemed gentle.

I liked gentle. I related to what he said earlier and asked him to be my partner. He agreed.

"Most people prefer to Dom or Sub, but for this exercise, you're going to try both," Rao said.

"I don't think I'm gonna like being a Sub," I said. It was the control thing again.

"We're a perfect match then. I don't think I'm going to like being the Dom," he said.

I was surprised, I assumed everyone wanted to be the Dom.

Rao instructed us to hold our partner's hands and look into their eyes.

The Irishman's were green with flecks of gold.

There was a lot of eye contact in this class. It was intimate. Probably more intimate than I'd been with anyone in months. It was nice. And too much.

As the Dom, I was supposed to use my eyes to communicate that he was safe. I did my best to send that message through eye contact and by rubbing his hand with my thumb.

My Sub held up his hands as I tied the rope around both of his wrists and tightened until I had the perfect knot. I admired my handi-work and also noted how beautiful the red rope looked against his pale skin.

"Subs, lower your eyes. You are no longer allowed to look at your Doms."

He lowered his eyes.

"Doms, make sure your Sub feels cherished. Reach up and stroke their face. Slowly."

I couldn't remember the last time I stroked someone's face like that. Yet here I was on an intimate level, stroking the face of a man I had met a few hours ago.

I couldn't even remember his name.

Tony?

Juvoni?

Alex?

I ran my thumb across his cheek, moving toward his bottom lip. I gently caressed it as his mouth opened in anticipation.

I crawled my finger up his face toward his ear.

I was starting to enjoy myself. The sexual tension was palpable.

"Subs, get down on your knees," Rao said. "You are in service to your Dom."

I followed Rao's additional instructions: holding the rope in one hand and restricting his ability to move his arms.

"Use your other hand to caress their neck and their collarbone. Make them feel safe. You are responsible for this person. They are trusting you with their body."

It was weird because this was the kind of thing that I thought I would hate about BDSM. An uneven exchange of power. Someone on their knees who wasn't allowed to look at me. I thought every bone in my body would be repulsed by it. I wasn't.

I was enjoying it. A lot. My lip curled into a feral snarl. My eyes hardened. I felt powerful and sexy.

My Sub leaned his body into my hand and moaned slightly.

"Do you like this?" I whispered.

"Immensely," he whispered back.

I studied him to see if it was a lie and when I saw he was enjoying it, I had a revelation. My partner *liked* being submissive. It turned him on.

Everyone took the role they wanted. It wasn't about stealing someone's power. It was about that person willingly giving it.

"Doms, raise your Subs to their feet. Look into their eyes."

His eyes were a darker shade of green, tinted by arousal.

Staring into his eyes I felt a lot of things too: arousal, compassion, power. Along with something else I couldn't identify, something that felt similar to aggression. It was something I had felt before, a primal urge to bite someone a little too hard. I quickly suppressed that one and focused on arousal instead.

"All right, switch roles."

I took a deep breath and scowled. I did not want to be the Sub. I didn't like anyone telling me what to do.

"Remember, being a Sub is an incredible gift. You get to surrender while someone else is taking full responsibility for your body and your pleasure. It's almost easier and more enjoyable to be a Sub," Rao said.

I wondered if that comment was related to my scowl.

The Irishman tied my wrists and pulled them behind my head. He was tentative and cautious about hurting me. I liked that. He was right; we were a good match.

I lowered my eyes, though I couldn't help but smile. He was trying hard to be the Dom. He was going through the motions but his gentleness permeated everything he did.

"Kiss your sub's cheek."

He cautiously lowered his lips to my face. His lips brushed my cheek.

"Run your hand down their arm."

As he increased the force of his hand, I tried my best to truly submit. I wanted to let him feel what it was like to really be in control. It was surprisingly easy but I think that was only because of his tenderness. I probably would have resisted if I had been with someone else.

I expected to feel helpless and weak. I didn't feel that at all. I didn't feel disrespected or lesser.

As I got down on my knees, he ran his hands over my shoulders, powerfully massaging me. In that moment, I felt exactly how Rao had instructed the Dom to treat the Sub—cherished. With every caress of his hand, the Irishman made me feel like he loved touching me.

"This is what good BDSM looks like," Rao said. "Too often it's one person getting what they want. A Dom spanking their Sub out of anger. That's not a game that ends well for anyone. Both parties must consent. Both parties must get what they want."

He was full of gems. He was like the Gandhi of dominance. The Mother Teresa of bondage. The Oprah Winfrey of leather.

The exercise ended and the sexual tension in the room was noticeable. I had never been in a space that sexually-charged. I felt certain that some couples were going to sneak away and have sex on the next break if they could.

We headed back to our seats. One of the class assistants grabbed me on my way.

"I was watching you during the Dom exercise. You're sexy. If you ever wanna go with me to a dominatrix den, let me know. There's plenty around the city," she said.

I laughed.

I wasn't exactly sure what one did at a dominatrix den, but whatever it was, I probably didn't belong there. They'd see right through me. I'd probably trip the alarm at the door and get kicked out before I even walked in.

Then again, I guessed I shouldn't rule it out. I'd never thought I'd be at a BDSM workshop in the first place.

The final lesson for the class was focused on spanking. As Rao went over the rules, I found myself zoning in and out. It had been a long and emotional day. It was a full-day workshop and despite the arousing subject matter, I needed another cup of coffee. I grabbed a cookie instead and returned to my seat to jot notes, yawning the whole time.

Rao called up one of his assistants, Ramona, for the demo. She was tall, six foot five, with a commanding presence. Completely naked, she strutted to the front and leaned over the table, ready to be spanked. She was a foot away from my face and her vulva was visibly wet. Rao demonstrated how to cup one's hand and pulsate the movement.

I winced as he increased the intensity. I didn't like it. It felt anti-feminist or something.

When the demo was over, another woman asked, "I can see how this is enjoyable for him, but how is it enjoyable for *you*, Ramona?"

Ramona laughed. She stood up to her full height.

"Well, to be honest, when I get spanked, I feel pain and a little bit of humiliation. Fear. Danger. I love that. Those feelings turn me on."

Her answer was clear, articulate. Once again, I was forced to question my own preconceived notions. I had ill-formed ideas about what it meant about someone's psychological state if they liked to be spanked or liked spanking someone. The truth: It didn't *mean* anything. It turned her on, simple as that.

Now it was our turn.

I wanted to work with the cute Irishman again but the guy sitting next to me asked first. I didn't want to hurt his feelings so I said sure.

We moved to a corner of the room and debated who would go first, until we settled on me.

"Are you gonna keep your pants on?" he asked as everyone else in the room was disrobing.

"Yes," I responded, aggressively enough that the couple next to us laughed.

I leaned against a chair and stuck my ass out.

Within thirty seconds I realized that, unlike Ramona, I was not into this.

"Try moving here. Faster. Never mind. Do this," I instructed.

He was right, it was hard to feel anything through my jeans but I refused to take them off.

"Shhh. You're supposed to be the Sub," my partner whined.

Oh yeah. I forgot. That's why I wasn't a very good Sub.

My mind wandered back to the beginning of class when Rao had said, "You shouldn't do anything you don't want to do."

Smack. My partner was spanking me a little too hard.

I wasn't enjoying it, but I was going through the motions to spare his ego. Rao was right, I shouldn't be doing that.

"I'm not really feeling this," I said. "I want to stop."

"Are you sure? Maybe if I . . ."

"It's not my thing," I said, kindly, but firmly.

We switched roles. Maybe I'd enjoy it more if I was doing the spanking.

I tried spanking him a few times before realizing that I really wasn't into that either.

We stopped, which gave us an opportunity to watch everyone else.

Most people were in their underwear. The Metamucil woman was totally naked and getting spanked by the "I want fuck you" guy from the shame exercise. Her face was contorted in pleasure. She was moaning loudly.

The sexy dark-skinned man was getting spanked and Dom'ed by a beautiful woman. He too looked like he was enjoying himself. A few people were fully clothed and chatting. I guess spanking wasn't for them either.

I spotted the Irishman and walked over to him.

"Don't like spanking?" I asked.

"Nah, I'm not interested in it."

I smiled. He was sweet. In a different phase of my life, I'd probably have gotten his number but I had too much to process from the day to even think about going on a date with anyone.

I was deep in thought when a man approached. I hadn't seen him earlier.

"Hey, you're Olive? I'm Sheng. Thought I'd drop by at the end, say hi to some friends."

Sheng was younger than I expected, maybe twenty-four or twenty-five with wavy, wild hair.

How could someone so young be a sex coach? I wondered.

He had an air of seriousness about him and intense, dark eyes.

"This was amazing. Thanks for inviting me."

He asked me how the rest of my adventures were going and when I told him I didn't have anything else planned, he said, "If you ever want to try OM'ing, let me know." He handed me a business card with his name written in gold embossed letters.

I folded the card carefully and put it in my pocket.

Everyone finished spanking and we all took our seats. While Rao was taking questions, I was reflecting on the day.

Everything I believed about BDSM had been wrong. I wondered what else I had gotten wrong.

I made a decision then and there.

I was all in.

I was going to spend the next year doing everything I could to learn about sex and I was going to write about it. Maybe I was a sex writer after all.

I knew that somehow, in a way I didn't fully understand, I'd reached a turning point, a life-changing fork in the road.

This was just the beginning.

OM'ING

Two weeks had passed since the BDSM class and Sheng's business card was sitting on my desk, untouched. The gold embossed card stood out among a surplus of pens and loose change.

I picked it up and turned it over in my hand, running my fingers over the tiny, metallic letters.

Like any good student, I'd googled OM'ing. I'd watched videos, read articles, and researched the company, OneTaste, a premier advocate for the practice.

If there was one thing I was really good at, it was academic learning. I did my motherfucking homework.

I learned that Orgasmic Meditation was a structured ritual that involved stroking the clitoris for fifteen minutes. It was a process that was meant to be spiritual and meditative. There were rules. Steps.

If there were a written test, I would have passed with flying colors with time to spare at the end of class.

Unfortunately, I knew this couldn't be academic. If I wanted to fix my sex life, it wasn't enough to browse the Internet. This year was about facing some of my insecurity around sexuality and the only way I was going to do that was by pushing myself out of my comfort zone.

One website claimed that OM'ing allowed people to "activate their sex impulse." I liked that idea because I was deeply concerned that mine was broken. Instead of pheromones, it was releasing a penis-repellent that smelled like desperation and loneliness.

I picked up my phone and texted Sheng to schedule a session.

"Hey, it's Olive! I'd like to take you up on your offer."

My friends in the sex-positive community informed me that OM'ing was old news; it had been written about in the *New York Times*, *Cosmopolitan*, and the *Huffington Post*. In some circles, I was late to the game.

Everyone else thought I was nuts for inviting a near perfect stranger to come over and rub my clitoris for fifteen minutes. The entire practice was focused on female pleasure, which made some of my friends, both male and female, ask, "What's in it for him?" Many of them thought it was a ruse to get me to have sex with him. I didn't think so. In many of the videos I watched, the men proclaimed that they loved OM'ing as much as the women. My friends couldn't comprehend why a man would give without getting anything in return. If I were a psychologist, that might have inspired an interesting study about how we're socialized to think about sex.

But I'm not a psychologist, thank God, so I didn't have to analyze those questions.

Then again, who knew? Maybe he'd come over and we'd be madly attracted to each other and I'd end the dry spell. I can't say it didn't cross my mind.

———

We scheduled the session for an afternoon while my roommates were gone. I had told them about it but had failed to mention that I was planning on using my roommate's room, which was much larger and cozier than mine.*

I was sitting on the living room couch in my fuzzy fleece pajamas, sans makeup, hair in a braid when the doorbell buzzed.

I hadn't tidied up my apartment or my vagina. I was intentionally trying to keep it as casual as possible. Looking nice meant I wanted impress him—which maybe I did, just a tiny bit; I just didn't want him to *think* I was trying to impress him or that I thought this was anything other than an OM'ing session.

I opened the door to find Sheng dressed equally as casually in sweatpants and tennis shoes, his wild hair a stark contrast to the intensity of his eyes.

"Olive, good to see you again," he said, extending a handshake.

"Likewise. Come on in! I was thinking we could, um, have some tea first and talk about what's going to happen," I said.

"Excellent idea," he said.

I motioned him toward the couch and ran into the kitchen to grab two mugs.

I returned, sat down across from him, and waited for him to initiate the conversation.

When he didn't, and I couldn't take the uncomfortable silence anymore, I said, "Do you mind if I take notes?"

"Of course not," he replied.

I jumped off the couch and ran to my bedroom to grab my green spiral notebook.

---

* Mary: Oh boy, this is awkward. If you're reading this, I owe you a nice dinner for this one. Red Lobster for some cheese rolls or something?

Given that he was a sex coach, I had expected him to be charming and flirtatious. Instead, he seemed a little awkward, which was making me feel more nervous than I already was.

I returned, flipped open to a blank page, and said, "So, how does this work?"

"Well, it's a process. There's an order to things," he said, explaining the steps in a linear fashion. His tone was formal and his vocabulary was textbook-y. He used terms I didn't know like "vaginal introitus."

I felt like I was at a doctor's appointment. Any thoughts I had about this turning into something more than OM'ing quickly dissipated. He was a professional.

I was surprised by the detail of each step and how every step had a name. Where I might say, "Shove a pillow under your butt and put a towel down so things don't get goopy" someone else had elegantly named the first step "Building the Nest." I wondered if somebody in the branding department at OneTaste had sat around a table brainstorming names before leaping out of their seat and yelling, "I've got it! We'll call it a nest."

After the Nest was "Grounding," "Noticing," "Stroking," "Grounding" (again), "Framing," and finally cleaning up the Nest.

It was, by design, thought-out and carefully planned. There was no room for creativity. Every detail was covered, down to how and where the stroker should sit.

I wrote each step in my notebook, underlining the names. Despite Sheng's thorough description, I still didn't get what the endgame was.

"What's the goal? Like, what if I don't orgasm?" I asked.

"That's the point. There is no goal. OM'ing is about teaching you to focus on the sensations in your body. It doesn't matter if you orgasm or not. That's what makes it meditative.

"Are you ready?" Sheng asked.

"Yeah . . . totally . . . Cool. Cool. okay, yeah. Let's do this," I said, hopping off the couch, starting to question what exactly I had signed up for.

I ran to my room to grab the pillows, towel, and blankets and brought them back to my roommate's room.[†]

We made the Nest by placing a blanket on the floor, with a pillow beneath both my head and my knees. Sheng placed another pillow by my right side for him to sit on.

"Cool. Cool. We're doing this," I said giving myself a pep talk. I lay down hastily, fully dressed, on the blanket, waiting for him to start.

"You might want to take your pants off," Sheng said with a hint of a smile, the first I had seen all day.

"Oh, duh, guess that's necessary," I said, standing up to remove my pants and underwear.

Sheng sat down on his pillow, setting the timer for fifteen minutes, the mandated time for the whole process.

Sheng followed the OM'ing rules by placing his left leg over my waist and his right leg under my knees to ensure that we both were in the most comfortable positions available.

He rubbed his hands together, warming them, before placing one firmly on my thigh. Using both hands, he massaged my bare legs, his muscles tensing and relaxing with each movement. This was the "Grounding" step.

He checked the timer.

"We're going to move on to Noticing."

---

† Hey Mary, at least I used my own linens. That counts for something, right?

"Noticing" meant that Sheng was going to describe the color, shape, and size of my labia and clitoris in detail. I had no idea what anything in or around that area actually looked like. The only times I had ever taken a mirror down there were the few times I thought I might have an ingrown hair.

I thought of adjectives people used to describe a vagina and came up with a short list of "flower-like," "roast beef," and "juicy," so basically the same list as a fifteen-year-old boy.

As for a clitoris? I had no idea how someone described it. Was mine long and oval? Pleasantly plump like a blueberry? Was it salmon pink or dirty-brown pink or not pink at all?

How did I not know what any of this looked like? Was I that out of touch with my own body? Would other women have an entire list of adjectives ready to go or was everyone as confused as I was?

I was so distracted by my own internal dialogue about the possibilities for describing a vulva that I missed Sheng's actual description of mine.

After "Noticing" came "Stroking," the part where Sheng actually touched my clitoris.

He put on a pair of milky latex gloves and opened a container of lube, placing some on his index finger.

As described earlier, he placed a finger at the opening of my vagina (turns out that's the vaginal introitus) and stroked upward before arriving at my clitoris.

He pulled back my clitoral hood, which I didn't even know was a thing before he told me, and placed his finger on the left side of the clitoris. The rules had been very clear that stroking happened on the LEFT SIDE ONLY. I had written it in my notebook in all caps. Apparently, there were more nerve endings on the left side.

He rubbed my clitoris unhurriedly, up and down.

Up and down.

Up and down.

Repeating the same motion over and over again.

Despite the fact that I was naked and a man was touching my clitoris, I wasn't aroused. He was a stranger and my body wasn't responding, so despite the lube, the friction felt painful.

My mind was racing with distracting thoughts, wondering how my vagina compared to other vaginas.‡

I should have shaved, I thought. Because even though it "wasn't an intimate experience," I still wanted to have an impressive vagina. This guy had seen a lot of vaginas and I wanted mine to be at least in the top five, even though I had no idea what would make a vagina "impressive."

Once I was done shaming my hairy vagina, my mind wandered to the voices of the Spanish-speaking ladies next door watching a telenovela. I could hear their conversation clear as day through the thin New York City walls and wondered what they would think if they knew what was going on next door.

As if reading my mind, Sheng said, "Where are your thoughts? Focus on what's going on in your body. Bring your attention to the sensation in your clitoris."

It was a much-needed reminder because I had been thinking about everything but that.

Focus on the sensation. Don't let your mind wander. This is meditative, I said to myself. I tried to bring my attention fully on my clitoris.

As I focused on heat flooding my body, it started feeling pleasurable. The sounds of my neighbor's soap opera were drowned out by my own

---

‡ Let's just get this out of the way. Technically the vagina is the canal on the inside and what can be seen on the outside is the vulva. I use them interchangeably a lot. But just to be clear, that's wrong. Be better than me and use the right terminology.

soft whimpers, which were partially authentic and partially to convince Sheng that I was enjoying the experience.

I still couldn't totally focus on the sensations because I knew the timer was ticking. Even though the goal wasn't cumming I wanted to get off. I was racing the clock. No matter where my body was, Sheng was going to stop after fifteen minutes.

"Hurry up. Hurry Up," I urged my body. *"You got this. Relax. Focus on the sensations and then you'll cum."*

It reminded me of countless times in college when I'd feel guilty about a man going down of me for "too long." I'd worry about his jaw hurting or his tongue going numb so I'd urge my body to reach climax ASAP, which usually resulted in a mediocre orgasm.

I imagined the army of women he'd OM'ed with before me, all beautifully orgasming at the exact right time from their perfectly groomed vaginas. I wanted to cum not just for me but also because there was a sense of pride in orgasming, like an orgasm meant that my body worked "right" and that was somehow "good."§ It was a fucked-up way of thinking about it but I still wanted to prove something to him (myself?).

The moans, although still soft, became more frequent.

I estimated that I had two minutes left until the clock went off.

Cum or bust.

I shifted my body upward until finally, with an estimated thirty seconds on the clock, I orgasmed, softly. It wasn't a great orgasm but I didn't care; I had beaten the clock.

As I was silently patting myself on the back, the alarm buzzed a minute later and Sheng began the Grounding process. He used his palms to put subtle pressure on my labia and thighs.

---

§ Is this why sex becomes "performative"?

We then had to describe the experience by saying things like, "When you _____, I felt _____." This was called "Framing." Sheng had no trouble with this part of the exercise.

"When you orgasmed, I felt a sensation of heat and electricity shoot up my arm," he said.

I wasn't as smooth. "Um. When you . . . did that . . . I felt . . . good."

He encouraged me to come up with a better description, but I couldn't so I just plagiarized his and slightly rephrased it. "When I orgasmed, I felt a . . . umm . . . pulsating and a rise in temperature."

It was total bullshit but I couldn't come up with anything else, so he let me off the hook.

I stood up and put on my pants.

I felt like we should hug or something but instead we headed back to my living room and sat on the couch.

"So, that's OM'ing. Do you have any questions?" Sheng said.

"How very interesting," I said, laughing at the fact that we were still being elaborately formal. We had just shared this intimately "non-intimate" experience and I wasn't sure how to process that.

I made more tea and sat down on the couch next to him, fiddling with the string from my tea bag.

Part of me wanted him to leave.

Part of me felt like I hadn't gotten the full experience because I was too nervous and too in my head.

Before I could chicken out I said, "Wanna do that again?"

Asking to OM was encouraged and supported in the OM'ing community so I knew I was being appropriate . . . and also a total greedy guts.

"Sure, you mean like another time?"

"I mean right now. I mean, we don't have to. I just think I need more research. I was too nervous the last time to really be fully immersed in OM'ing."

"Sure, happy to."

We headed back into the bedroom where we had left the Nest still fully assembled. I smoothed out the blanket and took off my pants and underwear quickly.

This time I was more relaxed from the get-go. I had already practiced the art of focusing on the sensation in my clitoris. My thoughts were fixated on the warmth I felt every time Sheng stroked me.

This time around there was no pain, only pleasure as Sheng stroked his finger up and down, steadily and evenly.

I moaned, 100 percent authentically. Loudly.

Bucking my hips slightly, I urged him to go faster and increase the pressure.

"Don't do that," he said firmly. "If you want me to do something, verbally communicate it. That's part of the exercise too. Say what you want."

I hated being rebuked but could acknowledge that it was a logical exercise. Thus far, a lot of my sexual communication was non-verbal. If I wanted something, I'd move my body a certain way or just do it myself. I was trained by the school of "Everyone is a mind reader and should somehow be able to figure out what they're doing."

"Faster," I mumbled.

He stayed steady and then increased both the pressure and the speed. He was a pro, I didn't need to communicate anything else.

I moaned louder, the sensation unlike anything I had felt in a long time.

I was about to have an intense orgasm. The Spanish-speaking ladies next door stopped talking. I should have been quieter but I didn't care. I was too engrossed in my own pleasure. In that way, I understood how it was meditative.

"Oh my God," I screamed. Followed by a breathless series of "holy shits."

My entire body spasmed and a flood of fluid gushed from my vagina. It was one of the most intense orgasms of my life.

Sheng went through the grounding and framing exercises before getting up and going into the living room. I lay there for a few minutes, panting and breathing heavily before putting my pants back on. I glanced at my reflection in the mirror in the hallway: my face was flushed and red.

Sheng was sitting on the couch casually sipping his tea.

"Wow," I said.

We sat silently for a few minutes. I wasn't sure where to go from there. That felt like nothing I'd ever experienced before. I wanted Sheng to leave so I could process and write about it.

Also, it was getting weird, pretending this wasn't intimate. He had just witnessed one of the wildest orgasms of my life and now we were talking about the new shoes he wanted to buy.

Finally, I said, "I'm sorry but I gotta leave to meet a friend in a few minutes."

Taking the cue, he said, "Okay, cool," grabbed his bag, and headed for the door.

"Can . . . Um . . . do I pay you now for the lesson?" I asked.

"I can't accept money or it becomes prostitution," he said with his signature matter-of-fact tone.

"Oh. Right. That makes sense," I said. I hadn't even thought about that.

I wasn't sure how to say goodbye, so I kept it simple and Midwestern: "Thank you so much."

"Anytime," he said, waving on his way out.

I walked back to my roommate's room and cleaned up the Nest, throwing the blanket over my shoulder.

I couldn't remember the last time I had been with a partner and had focused all my energy on the sensations in my body. All I had to do to elevate my orgasms was to bring consciousness to how my body felt. It was such a simple thing and yet it felt like a secret barely anyone knew about.

The OneTaste website boasted about the dramatic, life-changing power of the female orgasm. Renee had insisted that it was exactly what I needed to unblock my sexual energy.

She just might have been right.

For several days after OM'ing, I noticed a difference in the way I felt, as if was vibrating on a higher frequency and as a result, radiating happiness. People, especially men, were noticing. More people hit on me in the three days following my session with Sheng than in the whole rest of the month combined.

I was a non-believer. Until I tried it.

I couldn't wait to try it again.

THE STEALTHIEST EX

For the next three months I continued exploring sex in the best way I could think of as a single person. I went to classes, read books, and attended lectures. I became the Bill Nye of boning. My whole life was about sex.

Except I wasn't actually having sex. It was like learning to bake by looking at pictures in cookbooks.

What I really needed was someone to practice with.

Unfortunately, I was in a dead zone of potential candidates.

I wanted someone it wouldn't feel casual with, someone I trusted, someone who made me feel comfortable. Despite my best efforts I couldn't make a boyfriend magically appear in my life.

There was one person, though.

My ex, Mateo.

He was a sexy Italian who wore suits and planned salsa dates. When he looked at me, his eyes filled with lust. He loved my body, worshipped it almost. No one had desired me that way since. It had been three years since we'd dated, but we stayed in touch and occasionally grabbed lunch or coffee.

He had dumped me, out of the blue, via text.

Our failed relationship was the first time I realized I had some issues around sex. We had dated for six weeks but hadn't copulated* even though I wanted to. I was so worried that he'd want to try a crazy position and I wouldn't know how to do it. He'd write all over the Internet about his ex who couldn't figure out how to Corkscrew. His friends would comment on his post like, "OMG, seriously? It's not even that hard." He'd get drunk and tell his next lover all about my ineptitude. They'd go home and have passionate sex, pausing only once for her to say, "Bet your last girlfriend couldn't do this." He'd nod and they'd orgasm into bliss while I was home alone masturbating in missionary.

Every scenario ended with me being bad at sex and him dumping me, which was ironic because he dumped he anyway.

I had always felt like it was my fault it ended. If we'd had sex, or minimally if I had been honest with him about my hang-ups, things might have turned out differently.

After our breakup, Mateo was in and out of long-term monogamous relationships. When we met up there was always an undertone of sexual tension, but he was never a free agent, so nothing ever came of it.

Until one day I saw on Facebook that he was single.

It was my chance to right my wrong. I was one text away from breaking the dry spell, getting back together, and living happily ever after.

"Drinks tonight?" I texted him.

We planned to meet at a bar by my house.

He showed up forty-five minutes late, wasted out of his mind. He'd been at a basketball game earlier and drinking heavily since the afternoon.

---

* Have you ever tried to write a book about sex without using the word sex in every other line? It's hard!

He plopped down next to me on a stool.

"Hey sexy," he said going in for a kiss as if it was the most normal thing in the world even though we hadn't kissed each other in years. We both ordered beers and when we were finished with our first ones, I asked, "Want another drink?"

"No, I want you. Let's get out of here," he said, straightforward and to the point.

If it had been anyone else, I would have left immediately, but there was an element of trust that came from having a shared history. This sexual tension had been building for three years and finally, after all this time, we were gonna do something about it.

"Oh yeah?" I asked flirtatiously. It felt good to be wanted.

"Yeah," he leaned over to kiss me. He jumped off the stool and grabbed my hand, leading me out of the bar.

We walked quickly to my apartment and when we got inside, he threw his coat and bag on the floor. He made a quick motion to pull my jacket off before scooping me up and walking toward the bedroom.

Mateo had always been a good kisser but today his kisses were aggressive and sloppy. He undressed me and himself quickly and we fooled around until my serotonin and dopamine-soaked brain decided I was ready to end the dry spell, right then. Right there.

"Do you have a condom?" I asked.

"Um . . . no," he said, kissing my neck.

"Shoot. I might have one laying around," I said, jumping out of bed. I hadn't bought, used, or even looked at condoms in years, but luckily my roommate had one in her desk drawer.

I ripped open the packet and nervously unrolled it, trying to remember how to put it on correctly.

"You should probably do this," I said, handing it over to him.

He rolled the condom down his erect penis, kissing me passionately for a few minutes before reaching down to stroke my thigh with his hand.

I felt him rub the tip of his cock across me and he started to slowly enter. I could feel my muscles resisting because I hadn't had anything inside me for ages.

"Let me adjust. It might be more comfortable in a different position," I said, rolling around, pausing to kiss his stomach mid-roll.

Out of the corner of my eye, I glanced down at his erection. To my surprise, the condom was gone.

"Where's the condom?" I asked, assuming it had accidentally come off somehow.

He shrugged nonchalantly.

"I don't think I have another one," I said, pausing to kiss him deeply before jumping off the bed to rustle through my roommate's drawer again.

I returned to the bed empty-handed.

"No dice."

He shrugged again and made a grunting noise, before leaning in to kiss my shoulder and rubbing his cock dangerously close to me.

I pushed him away, annoyed. I was frustrated by the fact that we didn't have another condom but also by his breeziness. He didn't seem to be bothered at all.

"No condom, no sex," I said firmly. I didn't know his recent sexual history. If we were going to have sex, we needed to be cautious.

"C'mon babe, I'm clean. You know I get checked," he said, stroking my nipple.

Now I was pissed. I had no idea how often he got checked and I wasn't on birth control, something that he didn't know because he hadn't bothered to ask. I hadn't waited this long to break the dry spell haphazardly. I was a cautious person, and this felt reckless.

I sat up and folded my arms.

"I'm serious. No condom, no sex," I said.

"Babe . . . you're being unreasonable. It's fine," he said.

It wasn't fine. Not even a little.

"I'm not playing. We're not having sex without a condom. I'm not on birth control," I said.

I didn't owe him an explanation though. I thought we were using a condom, and suddenly there was no condom.

He sat up and stared at me.

I clenched my jaw and my fists, fuming. If he shrugged one more motherfucking time, I was going to lose my shit. Breaking the dry spell was a big deal to me. He was being careless and blasé about the whole thing, as if he didn't care if we had sex or not. Then he had the nerve to try to make me feel guilty about wanting to use protection? I wasn't experienced but even I knew that was wrong. It was such a pathetic disappointment after years of wishing Mateo and I'd had sex.

I lay down with my hands crossed over my chest and stared at the ceiling.

He made up some excuse to leave, and I was glad he did.

I walked him to the door.

"Bye, great seeing you," he said.

"Bye," I said as coldly as I could muster, letting the door slam behind him. I knew that was probably going to be the last time I saw him. I'd always assumed Mateo was an ex because we hadn't had sex, but maybe he was an ex because he was an inconsiderate asshole.

I raged for another twenty minutes before falling into a deep, angry sleep.

The following morning, when I woke up, one of my roommates, Lindsay was already awake, a large grin plastered on her face.

"Soooooooo, I ran into Mateo last night outside. Did you guys *finally* do it?" she asked.

"Nah, we didn't have a condom. Well, we had one, I mean one of yours, but then he lost it and we didn't have a replacement. Also, I owe you a condom," I said, grabbing a mug for coffee.

"What do you mean it got lost?" she asked, confused.

"Who knows. It was there and then it wasn't there."

"Hmm, that's . . . odd," Lindsay said with a concerned look on her face.

"What do you mean?" I asked.

She described an epidemic she had read about online called "stealthing" where a man secretly takes off the condom.

I stared at her in disbelief.

No way.

There was no way that had happened. It was an accident. An inconvenient accident but an accident all the same.

"Who would do that? That's . . ." I couldn't find the words. On a personal level, I placed such a high value on integrity that *that* level of dishonesty was unfathomable. Especially from someone I thought I could trust.

"There are forums teaching men how to do it. According to this article I read, it's alarmingly common."

"But what kind of piece of shit would do that?" I asked.

She bit her lip slightly before saying, "Maybe a piece of shit named Mateo?

"I mean, he *does* have a kind of shady history," Lindsay added, twisting her long, brown hair into a knot.

I started to refute this statement, but when I thought about it, I realized it was true. I had some serious revisionist history when it came to Mateo. I always painted him as a passionate man who adored me. The one who got away.

In my desire to make him seem great, I'd dismissed dozens of not-so-tiny red flags that had presented themselves while we were dating.

Suddenly I remembered other negative things about Mateo. Like how his best friend had cyberbullied me after our breakup. Like how his Halloween costumes were always offensive. Things he had said and done that pointed to the fact that maybe he wasn't the charming guy I wanted him to be.

Maybe the real Mateo was the kind of guy who removed the condom during sex.

I mentally replayed the events of the night before, analyzing the situation. It did seem odd that the condom had been there and then suddenly it hadn't been there, with no trace of it to be found, even in the morning. It also seemed odd how unconcerned Mateo had been about the whole situation.

I didn't know for sure how the condom came off, but the more I thought about it, the sicker I felt. I felt foolish and stupid for ignoring the warning signs.

I expressed my fears to Lindsay, who said, "You always see the best in people. It's one of your greatest qualities. You stood up for yourself in the moment with the knowledge you had. He's the piece of shit here."

I nodded. I didn't have time for jackasses.

Luckily, I didn't have too much time to think about it though because my roommates and I were in the process of moving . . .

. . . and I was busy falling in love with the boy in my room.

THERE'S A BOY IN MY ROOM

H is name was Adam Fansher.

He was my first crush after actively beginning my quest for coitus.

When I first moved to New York City I moved into a two-bedroom apartment with my friends from high school, Lindsay and Mary. In order to make city living affordable, I split a room and a bunk bed with Lindsay. We had been sharing a tiny closet and late-night chats, summer camp style, for almost five years. For the most part, I thought my bunking situation was hilarious, but six months before my thirtieth birthday, I knew I was long overdue for my own room.

Thirty and bunking?*

That was the kind of embarrassing story that went viral on Reddit. If I wanted to bone ever again, I needed a bed that didn't involve a ladder.

It was time to move.

We found a three-bedroom apartment in Harlem that we couldn't afford with a giant living room and natural light. I might have been okay financially if I hadn't been unexpectedly fired from my corporate

---

* In hindsight, it's super weird, but at twenty-five, we were just happy to be able to afford living in NYC at all.

job. I had somehow managed to get a job selling corporate training programs and over the course of one year, I had sold exactly nothing. I wasn't meant for sales, so I should have seen it coming, but I didn't. I had enough savings to cover one month's rent and after that I was royally screwed.

One week before my money ran out, God sent me Adam Fansher.

He had recently moved to NYC from Vermont and needed to sublet a room for four months.

I needed money.

I rented my brand-new room to Adam Fansher for extra cash. He slept on my bed while I slept on the living room couch. I hid my clothes in storage bins in our kitchen and hung my dresses in the hallway closet. It was a temporary solution until I could find a new job or get some freelance writing gigs. There was a four-month timeline. I told myself that anyone could live with anything for four months.

Not exactly how I thought my life was going to turn out.

My self-help books urged me to reflect on this. "What choices did you make to get here?" they'd ask. It was an excellent question that I didn't have time to ponder.

I was too busy living.

And too busy falling for the boy who lived in my room.

Adam Fansher was tall and lanky with a permanent five o'clock shadow and a mess of brown hair on top of his head. He ate three things: orange chicken, homemade pizza, and peanut butter sandwiches. He said the word "exactly" with an emphasis on the *T*. I'm not the kind of person who notices these things, which is how I knew I was falling for him.

He was gentle and spoke softly in a way that made it seem like he was really listening. He had a great sense of humor that was perfectly sarcastic without actually hurting anyone's feelings. He cared about the environment, was passionate about the arts, and went to see plays by himself. He wore sweaters that looked like they had been picked out by his mom. Whether it was due to proximity or chemistry, I wanted him in a way I hadn't wanted anyone in a long time.

Unfortunately, Adam Fansher was madly in love with someone else who'd broken his heart and moved to England. Her name was Jenny. He couldn't say her name without getting a little bit teary-eyed.

I knew it was a bad idea. I knew that emotionally unavailable people who were still in love with people who'd already broken their heart didn't have the capacity to be in love with me.

But I was too far gone. Heart and hormones were running the show.

Even though I knew he was sad over Jenny, I still thought there was something between us. We'd spend hours together: we'd meet up after work and go to the gym together and then ride the subway home together. We'd cook together, eat together. I looked forward to coming home because I knew that he'd be there. When he wasn't there, I didn't want to go out, in case he'd come home.

One Friday night, two months after he moved in, we decided to stay in and have a movie night. I curled up on my couch, under the blanket with my extra-large bowl of popcorn. Adam sat down next to me despite there being a perfectly open spot on the other end. He was closer than he needed to be with a lot of space to spare on his other side. It felt like a good sign.

We finished our first movie and agreed to watch a second one. It was midnight, the magical witching hour of flirting. Adam yawned, closed his eyes, and lazily laid his head in my lap.

Despite having lived together for months, it was the first time we had touched. I could smell the subtle scent of his body soap. I tentatively reached up and played with his thick hair. He made the human version of a purr.

My heart responded by beating rapidly.

I was aware of every part of his body. His head against my hand. His hair. His muscular arms.

He sat up and stared at me for a minute.

I licked my bottom lip, hoping he'd kiss me.

"I'm gonna head to bed. I'm tired," he said, standing up abruptly.

I wasn't sure what had just happened, but it was frustratingly anti-climactic. I watched him walk out of the room and laughed in confusion.

It made me want him even more.

My body was on fire.

I loved the chase and the buildup of sexual tension. The wanting to kiss someone badly enough that it becomes an all-consuming thought and when it actually happens it's electrifying.

I waited until I heard his door shut and settled in on the couch. I fantasized about breaking the dry spell with him while touching myself until I quietly came.

He was going to be worth the wait.

The next weekend, Adam and I spent our Friday night the same way. Movie. Popcorn. Hair stroking.

Followed by no kissing, going to bed, and solo masturbation.

Even though I liked the game, the sexual tension was becoming too much for me to handle. When was he going to make a move?

It felt like the fifth hour of playing Monopoly. I woke up horny and went to bed horny. I'd calm down and then see him in the kitchen, chopping onions in a cutoff shirt with his arm muscles rippling and I'd start all over again.

Something had to give.

My unquenched libido was manifesting in bizarre ways. I found myself sitting in a supermarket watching a man eat french fries, my pulse increasing as I watched his mouth close around the fry.

The good news was that my attraction to Adam was further proof that my sexual impulse wasn't broken after all. It was very, very turned on.

One night when Lindsay was wearing a T-shirt, I leaned forward and licked her arm, sloppily, like a dog. I didn't know why I did it except that I saw bare skin and wanted to lick it. The sexual tension with Adam was making me a total weirdo.

I needed to release my energy before I became even more desperate. Next, I'd wind up on *Dr. Phil* for randomly licking strangers on the subway.

Luckily, I had weekend plans to attend a birthday party. I couldn't do another going-nowhere movie night. I had to get out of the house. I spent a lot of time getting ready, picking out the perfect outfit and making sure I looked sexy.

"What do you think?" I asked Adam before leaving.

He whistled. "You look beautiful."

That was the whole reason I had gotten dressed up at all. I didn't care if my hair fell down or I tripped in a puddle after that.

I walked into the bar with an agenda: to kiss someone and get rid of some of the weird sexual energy I was harboring. Otherwise I was probably going to confess my adoration for Adam in an embarrassing fashion. I ordered a whiskey on the rocks with two ice cubes, knowing full well that whiskey makes me frisky.

An hour in and I felt magnetic. I was *on*. I scanned the birthday-party crew and saw some faces I didn't know, including a cute guy sitting on the couch alone.

I walked over to him and touched his hand.

"Anyone sitting here?"

"No, please." He gestured for me to sit.

"It's my lucky night. An open seat next to someone as handsome as you," I said.

I sat down, a little too close to him.

We chatted for a few minutes about how we both knew the birthday girl and how much we loved her before I touched his arm and said, "Are you single? I want to check before I flirt with you."

I knew I was being forward but I didn't care.

"One hundred percent single. And it's *my* lucky night that you decided to sit next to me," he said.

"Oh yeah?" I slowly took another sip of whiskey, looking at him seductively over the top of my glass. "Well then, how about you're my boyfriend for tonight?" I asked. I still didn't know his name.

"What does that entail?" mystery man said.

I could tell that he was intrigued, interested, and also hesitant. If I was looking for someone to date, I might have been a little less direct, but I didn't care if this man wanted to date me. I just wanted him to kiss me. I had nothing to lose by being fierce.

"I'm going to grab another whiskey and then I'll tell you. Wait for me. If anyone else asks, this seat is taken now," I said, strutting to the bar, surprised and impressed by my own confidence. I was never that bold.

It was fueled by whiskey and pent-up sexual frustration.

Usually I was the funny, sort-of-awkward sidekick type. Tonight, I was the Femme Fatale. The Leading Lady of Sexiness.

I walked back, second drink in hand.

"Where were we?"

"You were going to tell me what it meant to be your boyfriend for the night."

"Well we're gonna start with this . . ." I said, caressing his hand slowly.

"I like that," he said.

"What's next?" he asked, rubbing my arm with his other hand.

I scooched closer to him and said, "How would you feel about giving me a shoulder massage? All the best boyfriends give massages."

He rubbed my back sensually and slowly. It was precisely what I needed.

I was wearing an off-the-shoulder dress, which meant hand-to-skin contact. It was almost too much for my starving-for-touch body to handle.

"Should we talk about stuff?" he asked, pressing his thumb into a particularly stubborn knot on my back.

"What kind of stuff?" I asked.

"I don't know, but if you're gonna be my girlfriend for the night, we should probably talk about stuff." I turned around and smiled sexily, leaning forward until I was an inch away from his lips.

"I don't think that's necessary" I said, kissing him slowly and then more forcefully as the floodgates of my sexual dam started to burst at the seams.

I pulled away, but he leaned in and kissed me again.

"At least tell me your name," he said against my lips.

"It's Olive, yours?"

"Luke."

"Nice to meet you, Luke, boyfriend for the night," I said, kissing him again.

We made out for another ten minutes with very little talking before a friend who lived uptown by me approached us. "Hey, we're gonna get going. See you soon . . ." she said, implying that I was staying.

I didn't want to stay. If I got home early enough, Adam might still be up. Plus, I never passed up an opportunity to split a cab back uptown.

"I'm going with you," I said, standing up.

Luke looked dismayed. It was clear he didn't think that was how the evening was going to end.

"Bye, boyfriend," I said with a wink.

"Can I at least get your number?" he asked, confused. He handed me his phone and I added in my number before kissing him one final time.

By the time I got home, Adam had already gone to bed. I sat down on the couch and a text popped up on my phone.

"Hey, it's Luke. Nice meeting you tonight."

"You too." I texted back before falling asleep and dreaming about Adam.

Luke texted me the next morning and asked me out on a date.

We met for brunch the following week. Even though I was massively crushing on Adam, I didn't want to close the door on other possibilities. Especially possibilities who weren't in love with their exes.

I walked into the restaurant and saw Luke sitting at a table in the corner.

Even though we had already kissed, it seemed inappropriate to kiss him now. I gave him a hug and sat down.

We ordered food and made small talk for a few minutes before I realized that I knew nothing about him.

He was a science teacher and a movie buff. When I told him I was a writer, he told me I was going to make zero money. When I told him I was happy about losing my job and that I liked freelancing, he questioned my financial stability and commented on how hard it was to be a disciplined freelancer.

I felt like I had to be impressive and quite honestly, at that point in my life, I wasn't.

I was sleeping on my own couch, for God's sake.

This is why you should talk to someone before you make out with them.

Halfway through the date, we were struggling to find conversation topics.

At the end, he offered to walk me home. Even though it was blatantly clear that we had nothing in common, I let him hold my hand, because I was lonely, horny, and unrequitedly in love with the boy who lived in my room.

When we arrived at my gate he kissed me. I let him, for the reasons above.

"I'll text you," he said, even though I knew he probably wouldn't.

When I walked into my apartment, Adam was sitting on the couch in our living room reading a book. He had lit two candles and was eating a bowl of orange chicken.

"How was the date?" he asked, looking up from his novel.

It was an innocent question. On any other day I would have responded nonchalantly and moved on, but this time was different. The date was crummy, and it didn't even remotely matter because what I really wanted was the boy sitting across from me in my own house. My feelings were boiling over, and if I didn't say something I was going to explode.

"He kissed me," I said.

"Didn't you two make out at the bar the other night? What's the problem?"

It was now or never.

"The problem is that . . ." I paused to take a breath. "The whole time he was kissing me . . . I wanted to be kissing you," I said.

I could feel the blush spreading up my face. In thirty seconds I was going to be a deep shade of maroon.

He stayed silent as I turned dark red.

It felt unbearable, standing there visibly embarrassed. I didn't want him to see it, so I walked over to the light switch and turned it off, mumbling, "I don't want you to see me blush." Might as well be honest.

The room was lit by candles now, which might have been romantic if he was going to say something different than what he was about to say.

"I'm sorry, I can't . . ." he trailed off.

The silence hung between us and in it was everything I knew he wasn't saying. That he was still in love with Jenny. That he only saw me as a friend.

"It's okay," I said. "I needed to say that for me. I mean, it's not like I'm in love with you. It's a silly crush," I said, trying to diminish the situation.

Even though the room was dim I could see his eyes tear up. God bless him and his sensitivity; it was what I loved about him.

"I'm just . . . Jenny," he said.

"I understand, truly I do."

I did understand. It had taken me a long time to get over my own first love, and I still occasionally cried about him, more than a decade later.

"I'm a disaster. I can't date anyone. I don't even like myself right now," he said.

As he got more emotional, I felt calmer. Although I was the one being rejected, my self-destructive empathy kicked in and I felt the need to take care of him. If it was anyone else, I might have taken my moment to be angry and sad, but Adam was gentle and kind. It wasn't his fault that he didn't love me back.

"I value your friendship. I don't have a lot of friends here and you're . . . I just . . . I don't want to lose you," he stammered.

"You live in my house. You're stuck with me, kid, whether you like it or not," I said, gently.

"I don't want to hurt you."

"You're not hurting me. I'm a big girl," I soothed. "Let's watch a movie?"

He obliged, and, in some ways, it felt like every other night. In some ways it felt totally different. The sexual tension I had imagined for months was gone. I readjusted uncomfortably on the couch several times, hyper-aware of my body language. He avoided the couch and sat in a chair instead.

We said goodnight and nothing more was said about my confession.

For the next two weeks we were able to maintain relative normalcy, with occasional awkward moments. I was home less frequently and went out on Friday nights. We avoided any more movie nights. I went on dates and made sure to tell him about it. We both knew what I was doing, but it was a way of saving face. We still went on walks and I'd feel my heart twinge every time he said something funny, until I decided it was probably best we didn't go on walks anymore. When he asked, I made up excuses for why I was too busy. I wasn't heartbroken, but I wasn't a masochist either.

His four months were almost up. I didn't ask him to extend. I'd managed to save enough money to be more comfortable and I was tired of shoving my shit in the closet. I wanted my room back. Not to mention, my other roommates, who were total saints for going along with the arrangement in the first place, wanted the living room back.

Adam moved out and ended up subletting an apartment two floors above me, so I still occasionally saw him but I didn't come home to the smell of orange chicken.

I finally moved into my bedroom and for the first time in years, had a private room for conducting salacious activities.

My life could have become dangerously sexy. I could have taken my BDSM knowledge and everything else I was learning and put it all to good use.

I didn't, of course.

I felt like I was back at square one. No exes. No crushes. No prospects.

Single and alone as I had ever been.

THE MOST BEAUTIFUL PENIS IN THE WORLD

I didn't want to have casual sex.

That was the rule since the dry spell began. I hated the idea of going home with someone I didn't know or trust. Of waking up wanting to cuddle but uncertain if he wanted me to leave. I had a deep fear of being used.

From the beginning, I wanted to break the dry spell with someone I trusted. Someone who could possibly come along with a relationship.

Also, ever since I was a child, my paranoid father had convinced me that everyone was trying to kill me. When it came to my physical safety I was excessively careful.

"What if he's a serial killer?" I said to my friend Nathan after he suggested I go home with a random man eyeing me at the bar.

"Statistically speaking, how many people are serial killers?" he asked.

"ALL YOU NEED IS ONE!" I yelled dramatically. He rolled his eyes as I explained how I was saving my poor mother from a lifetime of grief.

Nathan wasn't the first to suggest this. Countless people proposed casual sex as the way to solve my problem. "Meet someone at the bar, go home with him, and just *do it*," they said.

But I didn't. Wouldn't. Because I was, down to the core, not interested in casual sex.

Until I took Ben home.

Then I was very interested.

I was still reeling from the debacle with Adam when my friend Erickson invited me out for drinks. Despite our seven-year friendship, Erickson and I couldn't be more different. He's vodka; I'm tea. He parties at expensive clubs while I watch TV in my jammies. He's the craziest friend I have. I'm the lamest friend he has. It made sense that he played a role in my first-ever one-night stand.

After not seeing each other for months, he suggested we meet up at a hotel bar with "a spectacular view." He loved pretentious, fancy places. I hated them. My Ohioan sensibility rejected the NYC socialite scene.

The hotel was luxurious with ceilings covered with chandeliers. The flooring was marble. Rooftop seating came with a lush red robe to ward off the cold while eating and drinking.

The maître d' glowered at us as Erickson requested a table for two for drinks.

"Tables are for food service. You can try downstairs," he said, dismissing us with a hand gesture. Downstairs, condescending employee number two informed us that tables were reserved for larger parties.

I scowled.

We turned to leave when a confident male voice with a sexy British accent said, "They're with me." I turned toward the source of the voice and was not disappointed when I found a boyishly handsome man sitting by himself.

I had never met this man. Neither had Erickson but he pushed past the maître d' to join the gentleman at his table, all of us pretending we were old friends.

"Are all Americans such jackasses?" the man asked with a hint of a smile after the maître d' left. "They wouldn't let me sit unless I was with a group. I'm traveling alone, so I told him my group was on the way. I'm Ben," he said.

Ben appeared to be about twenty-five. Despite being British, he had an all-American boy look, like a clean-cut model on an Abercrombie bag.

Erickson and I ordered drinks for our new friend, who turned out to be more culturally American than I was. Ben the Brit loved the United States. He played American football back home and preferred beer made in Cleveland. He thought American girls were sweet and funny. He liked burgers and fries. He was backpacking across the United States and was leaving New York in two days to make his way to the West Coast.

We had nothing in common.

He wanted to talk about football. I wanted to talk about anything else. We liked different music, food, and hobbies.

He wasn't smooth or overtly flirtatious like I expected him to be. On the contrary, he was shy and awkward. The only thing that kept the conversation going was our love of back-and-forth banter. When all other commonalities fail, it's amazing how far witty British humor can move things forward.

"I hate places like this. Let's go to a sports bar?" Ben said.

All right. We had one thing in common. I eagerly agreed, and we wound up at a generic sports bar down the street.

Ben bought the first round of shots.

I wasn't a big drinker, but I accepted because nights out with Erickson were some of my only "crazy" nights. Typically, I'd be asleep by midnight, a fact that was often brought up as a contributing factor in my coitus conundrum.

Erickson bought the second round.

Third round back to Ben.

The more we drank the more I was charmed by him. He was funny and the alcohol took away his shyness.

Drinks flowed until two hours later when Erickson announced that his booty call had contacted him and he was leaving.

Normally, I'd leave too.

Normally, I'd say, "It was nice to meet you. I'm heading out as well." Then I'd go home. Alone.

Maybe I was fueled by alcohol or Ben's sexy accent, but even I was surprised when I said, "I'm gonna stay."

Erickson cocked an eyebrow at me. "Don't do anything I wouldn't do," he said, smirking as he left the table.

"Another shot?" Ben asked.

With Erickson gone, I needed to be more cautious. I had met this man a few hours ago. After all, he *still* could be a serial killer. I imagined my mutilated body on the news with the newscaster saying, "They met at a bar three hours earlier."

My mom would be crying. "She never did things like that."

"I'll have a water," I said.

For having such different interests, we somehow managed to have a lively conversation for the next two hours.

Before I knew it, it was 1 a.m. and there were only two ways this evening could end:

1. We'd say "Goodbye, adieu. It was nice making your acquaintance, fair stranger." Ben would go back to his hotel. I'd go home. We'd never see each other ever again. The end.
2. The opposite of that.

I contemplated the situation, weighing both options in my mind. I tapped my finger on my lip, deep in thought.

"I'm not going to kiss you," Ben said leaning toward me.

"What do you mean?"

"You're tapping your lip like 'kiss me' and I'm not going to," he said, shaking his head.

How presumptuous of him. How utterly annoying. How even more annoying because I was, in fact, hoping he wanted to kiss me.

"Well, I'm not going to kiss you either. Not in a million years. Not even if—"

He cut me off mid-sentence by grabbing my face and kissing me.

"I couldn't let you keep going. A million years is a long time and I've been thinking about kissing you for a good hour."

His kisses were pleasant but not overly impassioned. He preferred short, quick kisses with less tongue. We kissed for a few minutes before he said, "Are we going home now or later?"

I was both impressed and annoyed by his confidence. Unfortunately, he had misjudged the situation. I wasn't the type of girl who went home with someone from the bar.

Then again, maybe I could be. I was tired of following meaningless rules that I had imposed on myself. Maybe I was too old-fashioned when it came to dating.

"No one buys the cow if they can get the milk for free," my long-standing guilt machine said to deter me. I couldn't, for the life of me, remember where I had heard that or why I had chosen to believe it.

Besides, that expression wasn't relevant here. Ben was leaving in a few days. There was no longevity in this. It wasn't going to turn into a relationship.

I kicked the can down the road and pretended not to hear his question. "How's that whiskey?" I asked.

"Good. But I'd be perfectly content leaving it here if I knew I was going home with you."

Now he was being too pushy.

"I'm not having sex with you," I said, finally making a decision.

"Who said anything about sex? I thought it would be nice to make out and cuddle."

I laughed. Like I hadn't heard that one before.

He must have seen the skepticism on my face because he added, "Seriously, make out and cuddle. That's it. Would be nice."

He was right, it would be nice to cuddle. Plus, his body was sturdy, and that British accent was sexy. There was something likable about him that made him seem sincere and safe.

"I'm serious though. I want to set the expectation. We're not having sex. I don't know you and I don't have sex with people I don't know."

He agreed, kissing me sweetly before grabbing my hand to leave.

For the first time in my life, I left with a boy I met at a bar, for no reason other than I wanted to.

Twelve subway stops later, we walked through my apartment door. I led him back toward my room.

We crawled into bed and spooned for a bit, neither one of us making any sort of move.

It took about ten minutes before his hand moved cautiously toward my rib cage, right below my left breast.

Even though I had mentally and verbally set the expectation, my body reacted to the closeness of an attractive male in my bed. I wanted him to move his hand upward. I shifted slightly until his hand rested an inch away from the curve of my breast, unmoving, his fingers twitching slightly. He was waiting for permission from me.

I felt conflicted because I wanted to "just make out" but also wanted him to touch me in a way that I knew was more than that. My fears about one-night stands were waging a war against my primal instincts.

Primal instincts won.

I grabbed his hand and placed it on my breast.

I rolled over and kissed him longer than he liked, trailing pecks down his neck before peeling off his shirt to reveal a toned and tan torso.

He pulled off my shirt and timidly tracked kisses down my stomach, arriving at the top of my jeans.

"I want to taste you," he said.

I should have been thrilled to hear that but instead it triggered an alarm in my brain. The caution I had thrown to the wind a few minutes earlier came back with a vengeance.

"What if he has oral herpes?" my inner voice said. Unlike Anastasia Steele's, my inner voice wasn't a goddess or even sexy. I wasn't even sure my inner voice was on my side most of the time. In my mind, my inner voice was a man. A snaggle-toothed, ex-pro wrestler who only wore cut-off shirts, to be exact. He was intense and always screaming at me.

"You're being paranoid," I told him, enjoying the kisses on my stomach.

"No! You're being reckless," he shot back. "It's all fun and games until this boy is long gone and your vagina is itchy."

Goddamnit. He had a point.

"You can't go down on me," I said to Ben. "Believe me, I want it to happen. It's not a good idea."

"Why not?" he asked, running a finger over my panties.

Because a crazy man in my head said so, I thought.

"Because I don't know you and your history," I said.

We continued making out and groping each other, the body heat intensifying with each movement. The sexual tension was culminating but I had no idea where it was going to end.

"If you want to have sex, we can use a condom, so you don't have to worry," he whispered against my collarbone.

I'd still worry. Because the snaggle-toothed ex-pro wrestler had once done a Google search that resulted in the knowledge that condoms don't always protect against STDs.

Google searches are bad for getting your mojo back.

My primal instinct for sex was duking it out with my overall general anxiety.

I kissed his stomach and pulled off his boxers.

Just like London's most iconic landmark, Ben was big.

Big was an understatement.

He was enormous.

Alarmingly large. If Michelangelo and Zeus joined forces to create a penis, it would have been Ben's.

It was also the most aesthetically beautiful penis I had ever seen.

There was no way in hell it was going inside of my vagina.

I hadn't had penetrative sex in five years. That thing was a beast meant for pornos and bachelorette parties.

Most women's eyes would have lit up with excitement at the sight of Ben's penis. I was scared. It was never gonna fit. Not comfortably. Not in a million years. Bigger wasn't always better.

I stared at it for a second, debating my next move.

I wanted to lick it, out of curiosity, to see what the world's most beautiful penis tasted like. I leaned my head forward and flattened my tongue against the base, taking a few inquisitive strokes from the base up to the head.

I licked a few more times before wrapping my lips around him.

Like clockwork, the ex-wrestler showed up, agitated. His muscles bulging. He looked furious. "What if he has genital herpes and now you're putting your mouth all over him? What are you thinking?!"

I wasn't thinking.

And it felt good.

Thinking was typically my problem.

I kept my lips wrapped around Ben's perfectly perfect penis, flicking my tongue across the head.

The wrestler tried again, "Hope it was worth it when your mouth is covered in sores."

He was the worst, always dropkicking me in the face.

He was right, though. I had just met this man a few hours earlier and although he seemed honest and sincere, I had no idea about his sexual history. I had no idea if he cared about my sexual health or not, if he'd had unprotected sex recently.

I removed my mouth and placed his fingers near my vagina.

We were both riled up and wanted to get off.

Fingers seemed safe.

"What if he didn't wash his hands?" the wrestler quipped.

Now he was being ridiculous.

I was too distracted to enjoy it until I remembered what I had learned in OM'ing. "Focus on the sensation and drown out the noise."

I told the ex-pro wrestler to shove it and focused on the feeling of his finger on my clit. It was the first time I was able to use something from my studies in a real-life scenario.

I'd be damned. It worked like a charm and before long I was orgasming from his touch.

We lay in bed for a few minutes before I got up to go to the bathroom.

Standing under the fluorescent light alone, I tried to enjoy the post-orgasm bliss, but my mind kept wandering to the wrestler and his premonition about my oral health.

I reached under my sink and grabbed a bottle of hydrogen peroxide. I poured it in a cup with water and gargled the mixture around my mouth for thirty seconds before spitting in the sink and then repeating the process all over again.

When it came to my sexual health and STDs, I was grossly undereducated. Like most people, I had turned to the Internet for information, which only caused increased paranoia.

I had absolutely no idea, evidence, or research that hydrogen peroxide would kill any germs Ben may have had but it calmed my brain a little.*

I stared at myself in the mirror.

Gargling hydrogen peroxide was insane. That wasn't a thing that normal people did.

I placed my forehead in my hands and shook my head. No wonder I was in a goddamned dry spell, I was out of my fucking mind.

I thought about my favorite book, *Catch-22*. One of the main themes is that if you're sane enough to realize you're crazy, then you're not crazy. According to that logic, I wasn't crazy. I fully acknowledged that I was behaving irrationally.

I brushed my teeth and headed back to my room.

While I was questioning my sanity in the bathroom, Ben fell asleep.

I crawled into bed. He stirred a little, rousing enough to kiss me before falling back asleep.

I woke up the next morning, groggy and glad we were at my place. I didn't have to worry about sneaking out or anything like that.

Ben woke up a few minutes after me. I assumed he'd make up some sort of excuse as to why he had to leave immediately. I thought all one-night stands ended with shitty mornings.

He surprised me by saying, "I'm hungry, wanna go get waffles?"

---

* I don't want to get on my soapbox here but can we please get some actual sex education in schools?! I'm the poster child for why we need it.

As we headed to breakfast, he held my hand and kissed me in the elevator.

"What are you doing tonight?" he asked at the diner, dousing his waffles in maple syrup. "I have one more day in NYC."

We met up again that night at a bar. We ordered drinks for each other and pretended to be a couple. He came over again that night. Ironically, this time we just cuddled. We were both too tired from the lack of sleep the night before to even attempt fooling around.

We grabbed breakfast again before Ben headed to the bus station to leave for good.

It was my first-ever one-night stand.

Almost.

Did it count as a one-night stand if we didn't have sex? I wasn't sure.

I walked into my apartment to find my roommates slow-clapping on the couch.

"Saw a pair of men's shoes by the door this morning, what's that all about?" Lindsay asked, smirking.

We had lived together for five years and I'd never brought a random guy home from the bar.

Ever.

I told them the whole story, including the part about gargling the hydrogen peroxide. I thought it was hilarious.

I could tell by the worried look on their faces that they didn't think so.

"You should go see a therapist," Lindsay said gently.

"Are you kidding me? C'mon. It's funny. I don't need to see a therapist to talk about sex. It's totally normal. I'm totally normal."

This had quickly turned into a goddamned intervention and I wasn't having it. Lindsay had recently started seeing a therapist and was convinced that it was a cure-all for everything.

Mary chimed in. "How do I say this kindly? You haven't had sex in almost five years and it seems like maybe you have an irrational fear of STDs."

"No, I don't. I think it's perfectly rational and even *smart* to be concerned about sexual health. Anyone would agree with me," I said.

Lindsay paused, carefully choosing her words. "We've been friends for fifteen years. And I've noticed that in the last five, you're a *little more* concerned than most people about STDs. You're not cautious, you're fearful, and it's affecting your relationships. You're amazing. You deserve to be loved, but there's something inside of you preventing that from happening. Listen, sometimes it's useful to talk to someone about the stuff that's going on in your brain," she said.

I sat silently for a second and thought about what they were saying.

Two days later, I called Dr. Rachel D'Souza, a sex therapist based in NYC.

ALL THE DEEP SHIT THAT IS
REALLY WRONG WITH ME

For years people had tried to psychoanalyze me, trying to figure out *why* I was in a dry spell. Lindsay and Mary had tried to lovingly armchair evaluate me as long as we'd been roommates. I'd get annoyed because, in my mind, I was totally fine.

I wasn't totally fine, though. Lindsay was right, there was some stuff that needed to be addressed, not by well-intentioned friends but by an actual therapist.

I began therapy after the Ben incident because I knew that I hadn't totally behaved like a rational human being.

If I wanted to fall in love or have sex ever again, I had to deal with my emotional baggage instead of pretending it didn't exist.

During our first Skype video session, Dr. D'Souza asked me about my childhood, past partners, and the dry spell.

We covered a lot of ground before I brought up my fear of STDs and what happened with Ben. I told her the entire story including the gargling of hydrogen peroxide.

She listened intently, her mouth curling into a soft smile.

"That's a quick leap to make. 'You are naked, I am naked, therefore I will get an STD.' It sounds like you're having irrational thoughts."

I laughed. *No shit*. That's why I was talking to a therapist. I wouldn't have called her if my thoughts were peachy keen and totally normal.

"Where do you think this fear came from?" she asked.

I knew exactly where it had come from.

I had been diagnosed with HPV when I was twenty and still a virgin. My gynecologist left a message on my voice mail saying that I had HPV and it was super common.

Also, the message said I had genital warts.

I had listened to the message in the front seat of my car in the Target parking lot as my whole body went numb.

I had genital warts.

My whole life, all I had ever heard was that people with STDs were "dirty" and that meant that you were "promiscuous." There I was, a twenty-year-old virgin with genital warts.

"What happened after you found out?" Dr. D'Souza asked.

What happened was that I lost my fucking mind.

Because I was young, and the health-care industry didn't know enough about HPV at the time, I took on horrible beliefs about what that meant for my future.

I convinced myself that no one would ever love me because my body was now a vessel for a transferable infection that no one wanted.

I had a few friends with herpes and most of them were in happy relationships. They knew that it wasn't a big deal, not really, and had made peace with themselves.

I couldn't.

I did awful things that I read about on the Internet to my body in an attempt to find a "treatment," like soaking tampons in apple cider vinegar and placing them inside my vagina. The more it burned, the more I convinced myself it was working.

I confessed this all to Dr. D'Souza with immense shame—that I had caused myself to suffer so much—and also anger. I was angry at my doctor for leaving a fucking message on my voice mail. I was angry at the health-care industry for spreading unnecessary fear about HPV, a virus that usually becomes undetectable. My voice was cracking the entire time, tears dripping down my face.

It was something I had never confessed to anyone, not even during the BDSM shame exercise. By confessing it all to Dr. D'Souza, it felt like I was showing her the parts that were ugly and twisted. I was terrified if anyone knew the truth or how crazy I went, they'd never see me the same way.

Dr. D'Souza nodded, encouraging me to go on. We both knew that, despite it being a difficult story to tell, I had to do it if I was ever going to heal.

I told her that two years after my original diagnosis, I made an appointment with a new gynecologist to have my genital warts frozen off.

During those two years I avoided dating. I'd go on first dates and call things off before I had to tell the truth.

As I drove to the gynecologist, I prayed on the way that somehow, by some miracle, this had all been a bad dream.

When I arrived, the waiting room was full of glowing pregnant women. The receptionist asked why I was there and when I said, "genital warts" my face turned red. Afterward, I avoided looking at any of the pregnant women.

My shame was eating me alive.

By the time my gyno called me back, I was just grateful to escape the waiting room.

While I lay there, dressed in a thin paper gown, my legs spread open, the gynecologist examined me for several minutes before speaking.

I assumed her silence meant it was bad.

After a few minutes she said, "What genital warts?"

I looked at her, confused, certain that I had heard her wrong.

"Honey, you don't have genital warts."

"What do you mean?" I asked.

She said it again, "You don't have genital warts."

"Wha . . . are . . . are . . . you sure?" I asked.

"I am 100 percent sure. Maybe you *had* genital warts at some point in time, but you don't now. Genital warts are caused by the Human Papillomavirus or HPV, and luckily, it's a virus that usually works its way out of your body in a few years. We're still learning about it but in most cases, both the HPV and the genital warts clear up on their own. I'll do a test for HPV but I'm willing to bet it's going to come back negative."

What?

HPV goes away?

Genital warts go away?

I had been carrying this around for two fucking years. I let it dictate my self-worth. I let it dictate who I believed would love me and who I thought I deserved, which was no one.

Still naked and shivering from the cold of the speculum, I began to cry deep sobs of relief.

As predicted, the test came back negative. I was tested six times during the next three years by four different doctors. They always came back negative for HPV with no signs of genital warts.

Finally, one of my gynecologists said, "Weren't you tested five months ago?"

"You can never be too sure," I replied.

She told me the guidelines had changed and the annual pap smear and HPV test was now recommended every three years. Studies had found that a positive HPV diagnosis was causing too much psychological damage to young women and, in most people, HPV was transient.

Or in other words, people were losing their fucking minds over an HPV diagnosis that would become undetectable.

I stared at her for a second, incredulous.

"I was one of those people," I said.

I was angry, again, at the fucking health-care industry. I was angry at myself for allowing my own diagnosis to grow and expand so deeply into my personal narrative.

That anger returned when I was talking to Dr. D'Souza.

She listened intently, letting me tell the story in its entirety.

When I was finished, she said, "That's very traumatic. I'm sorry you had to go through that. No wonder you're afraid."

I appreciated her empathy. It *was* traumatic, and I hadn't dealt with it, so it was creeping back into my life almost a-motherfucking-decade later.

"Wanting to be safe is rational and responsible. Feeling deep fear around STDs, using tampons with vinegar, and rejecting partners who have been tested is irrational. Do you see the difference? It's the same logic as this, 'If I go to gym, I will be healthier.' That's a rational thought. 'If I don't go to the gym, I will be unhealthy and die.' That's an irrational thought."

It was hard to figure out where the line was. For years, I had convinced myself that I was being cautious and that was smart.

If I was going to evolve as a person, I had to be honest with myself that my fear was crippling me.

I listened as she gave me a strategy to combat my fears. It involved a series of questions to get to the bottom of whether the thought was rational or not and then using logic to calm myself.

It seemed almost too simple.

I'm not sure what I was expecting, but I wanted to be "cured" of my fear around STDs. I wanted to get off Skype and immediately be better. "Hello world! It's me, Olive, totally fixed and ready for sex."

That's not how therapy or life works, so I wrote down Dr. D'Souza's questions skeptically and studiously.

We had a few more Skype sessions and I started to realize how far down the rabbit hole I'd gone.

Back when I had been diagnosed with HPV the Internet knew nothing about it except that it "was a virus that lasted forever," which obviously turned out to be false. A decade later, an Internet search revealed other women who had done similar things to their bodies. Women who had had parts of their labia removed. Women who had ended relationships or sworn off dating.

When I read these stories, I found strength in knowing how alone we'd all felt.

I also started forgiving myself for the things I had done when I was young and scared.

I promised that I was never, ever going to treat my body like that again.

Dr. D'Souza and I knew that talking about it could only go so far though.

I needed to test her strategies in action.

Luckily, I didn't have to wait too long.

Ben, the sexy Brit, came back to town.

He had finished his road trip across the United States and was flying home out of New York. He had three days to kill in the city before he left. We had stayed in contact while he was traveling. He'd send pictures of himself on a ranch in Texas and then later by Hollywood Boulevard.

We met up at another sports bar. He looked tanner and a few pounds heavier but still handsome.

"Turns out the prettiest American girl was the one I met first," he said when he saw me. Still a charmer.

He paid for dinner and held my hand. Even though we both knew he was leaving, it felt like a real date.

We met up the next night as well. After dinner, I invited him back to my place.

With great enthusiasm, we undressed and picked up right where we had left off.

We were on the verge of 69'ing when I felt the panic creep in. It was slow at first, just a thought, "What if he fooled around with someone on his trip and got an STD?"

The panic started at my brain, crept slowly down my arms and legs, and filled my feet and fingers until my body was merely a vessel for anxiety. It was the only thing I could think. *He's going to give me something and then he'll be gone.*

I squirmed away from him.

"Everything okay?" he asked.

What would Dr. D'Souza tell me to do right now? I thought.

First I had to check in with myself: Did I want to keep going?

The answer was yes.

Next step, ask a question to get the truth.

"Um, have you been tested recently? Like, did you fool around with anyone else on your trip?" I asked.

"I was tested before my trip and no, I didn't fool around with anyone else," he said.

I breathed a sigh of relief. I didn't realize I'd been holding my breath.

"Are you, um, sure?" I asked again.

"Sure, about being clean or fooling around with someone else?"

"Both?"

"I'm sure about both," he said.

"Because, like, honesty is very important. Are you absolutely sure?" I asked for a third time, fidgeting with my hair.

I could feel it. I was on the verge of jumping off a rationality cliff into a pool of panic.

After he confirmed for a third time, I excused myself and went to the restroom.

Even though his dick had only been in my mouth for a few seconds, I opened the white, chipped medicine cabinet and grabbed the bottle of hydrogen peroxide.

I looked at myself in the mirror and saw someone who was very, very afraid.

Afraid of intimacy. Afraid of tiny, invisible germs. Afraid of *living*.

The face staring back at me was sad.

My knuckles turned white as I clenched my hand around the bottle like an addict.

I didn't want to do this anymore. I couldn't do this anymore.

Other people weren't doing this.

I splashed my face with water and took deep breaths like Dr. D'Souza suggested. I imagined the questions she'd ask, playing out the dialogue silently in my brain, flushing the toilet at the same time so Ben wouldn't get suspicious.

"Is this a real fear?" she'd ask.

"Maybe, if your partner is lying," the wrestler chimed in, back in full force, veins bloated and expanding by the minute. It was his final attempt to ruin my life.

I unscrewed the cap on the bottle.

I wasn't going to let him win. I imagined Dr. D'Souza asking me again, calmly, "Do you believe your partner is lying?"

"No," I said firmly, out loud.

"Then is this a rational fear?"

"No."

I screwed the cap back on the bottle.

I looked at myself in the mirror again and repeated, "I refuse to let irrational fear run my life." I said it over and over again until the message started to sink it.

I placed the bottle on the edge of the sink and took a few more breaths.

I was finally able to calm myself down, not because of the technique but because I didn't want this to be my story anymore.

I was tired of being the girl who was terrified of STDs.

I was done.

I *had* to be done.

I returned to the bedroom slowly, trailing my finger down the wall as I walked.

"Sorry about that," I said, crawling back into bed with Ben.

"Now, where were we?" I asked, leaning in to kiss him.

We fooled around this time and instead of fear, I let myself feel pleasure.

We still didn't have penetrative sex though. Baby steps.

With Ben's arm around me, post-orgasm, I listened to his light snores and realized I had done it.

I had faced my fear of STDs.

I had finally worked through my shit and was ready to be a fully functioning erotic goddess with no issues. Come at me boys!

Yeah, right.

But I *had* successfully taken action against my fear at least once. That counted for something. That was progress.

Like I said, baby steps.

FETISH FERVOR

The Queen of the Foot Fetish Scene was a petite redhead with a firm handshake and a bubbly smile.

I met her at a trendy coffee shop in Midtown Manhattan. Even though it was our first time meeting, I had already seen a man devour an ice cream sundae off her foot. Whipped cream, chocolate sauce, and the works dripping between her toes.

Her name was Barbie Berdini and she was basically the Kim Kardashian of feet. She had created a foot empire. Her YouTube channel (where I had watched the aforementioned sundae-ing) was immensely popular. It was filled with videos of her feet in silky nylons or flip-flops, toes always perfectly pedicured. Sometimes she'd seductively crawl into the room, or the camera would focus on her butt before moving in for a close-up on the bottoms of her feet. Even though it wasn't my thing, there was no denying that she was stimulating.

Her fans wrote comments about how she was a "goddess" and "an angel baby from heaven."

No one ever called *me* an angel baby from anywhere.

In between my gut-wrenching therapy sessions I was still learning about sex and I was fascinated by fetishes. I had never given myself permission to explore or even fantasize in that way. After the BDSM class, and how fun it had been to dominate, I wanted to see if I was into anything else kinky.

Foot stuff had never been on my radar in any sort of sexual capacity.

I've had gross feet all of my life. Dry, cracked. At a party in tenth grade, a boy offered to give me a foot massage, saw my feet, and said "Yo, nevermind." I've kept them covered ever since.

Despite my own foot calamity, feet are one of the most popular fetishes.

I wanted to know why.

So here I was, with the Divine Foot Goddess herself.

Barbie ordered a cappuccino, I ordered a coffee, and we sat down, surrounded by businessmen in suits, to discuss the very serious matter of licking a toe.

Barbie was wearing jeans and a pink T-shirt with a cartoon picture of her face above the words "The Barbie Show." Her bright red hair matched her red lipstick. She was wearing sneakers and appeared to be about my height, no taller than five feet.

I had only seen her wearing sexy outfits and stiletto heels, so I was disarmed by the casualness of her appearance. "Thanks for meeting with me!" I said.

"Of course!" She smiled brightly, full of warmth and energy. I could already tell we were gonna be friends.

Before I could barrage her with questions, Barbie adjusted her chair, moving her feet away from me. "I'm sorry if it's smelly. I'm prepping my socks for resale," she said.

I sniffed the air subtly but couldn't smell anything but burnt coffee and macaroons.

"You're prepping your socks?"

She clarified: "I sold these socks for a hundred and fifty dollars. The buyer wants the socks to smell like my feet, so I have to wear them around for a few days before shipping them." She said it with a glint of good humor in her eyes, acknowledging that it was unusual without being apologetic.

Ironically, Barbie was sitting underneath a purple and pink poster that said, "Follow Your Passion." She had done just that, and now she was selling her socks on the Internet for a hundred and fifty bucks.

If I were sitting underneath a poster it would have said, "Still Figuring Shit Out." I thought of all the trips to the laundromat and sighed. To think, all these years I could have been selling my old dirty socks.

"Also, I swear I don't always wear a T-shirt with my face on it. We're filming new episodes for our YouTube show tonight," she continued, smiling.

I was impressed. Like the rest of us, she was grinding away trying to build her empire. She was the Queen not only because she was beautiful but also because she was a smart businesswoman.

I wanted to know how someone became the Queen of the Foot Fetish scene. I imagined her right out of college, wearing a suit from H&M and sitting in a bland corporate office. One day, after an unproductive meeting, she shoved all the papers off her desk and yelled, "Screw you! I'm ALL IN on feet!"

But Barbie was easygoing and down-to-earth. She didn't seem like the paper-flinging, screaming-as-she-exited kind of gal.

"So, how did you get into all this?" I asked, taking a sip of my coffee.

She smiled, pearly white teeth contrasting the dark lipstick.

"Well, one of my first boyfriends liked feet and I realized that I did, too," she said.

She told me a story about how they explored the fetish together in the backseat of his car and she realized how much feet turned her on. Even after their breakup, she continued to explore with her next partner.

Halfway through her story, the woman sitting next to us glanced up, obviously intrigued. She pretended to continue reading her book, but I could tell that she was still listening, mesmerized like I was by Barbie's candor.

"What do you like about feet specifically?" I asked.

I couldn't think of a single reason to like feet beyond functionality (they helped me walk, stand, do yoga). Lips were kissable and wet. Hands were smooth and soft. What redeeming qualities did feet have?

Apparently a lot.

Barbie liked the way they felt (smooth and wrinkly). She liked the way they tasted (sometimes sweaty, sometimes like soap, sometimes like skin). She and her community of foot worshippers loved the feeling of a foot smushed against their noses. She described the smell of a sole with the same fondness I'd use to describe a freshly baked blueberry muffin.

Before I met her, I was expecting this to be a farce. I thought perhaps she was someone who had capitalized on an underrepresented industry. She'd show up and be like "Look at me, I make money making videos of people licking ice cream off my feet. What a bunch of suckers!" That wasn't the case. Not only did Barbie sincerely have a foot fetish, but she also loved her job. She spoke about her fans with a sense of gratitude and loyalty. Her mission in life was to end the shame around sex and destigmatize fetishes.

I was on board with that.

Licking a foot seemed pretty harmless.*

---

* The irony isn't lost on me that licking a dick sent me into a downward hypochondriac spiral. But feet? Nah, totally fine.

At the exact moment Barbie was gushing about her fans, an older gentleman in a dark gray suit walked in and did a double take when he saw her. He pulled out his phone, looked at it and then back at her.

Barbie turned, smiled at the man and winked.

I had been so intrigued by the conversation that until now, I hadn't noticed that another younger man across the café was also sneaking glances at Barbie.

As I scanned from one man to the other, it occurred to me that I was having coffee with a quasi-celebrity.

I straightened my posture.

"I know you make videos on YouTube and sell your socks, what else?" I said.

"Oh, I haven't told you about one of the best parts, Barbie's Boutique! It's a luxury experience where people can either have their feet worshipped or come and worship one of my girls' feet."

"You have girls? Like, you're a madame?" I said, casually relaxing my hands behind my head.

"I wouldn't use that terminology, but yes. I organize everything with my team, make sure my models are safe, and review the rules with clients," she said.

"And then people pay . . . to what?"

"It's usually a customized experience for the client, but typically I'd say they spend an hour with their model, massaging their feet, licking their toes. Stuff like that," she said.

Anticipating my next question, she added, "And yes, it's all legal."

"But, like, it's just feet?" I asked.

"It's all foot and foot-adjacent. Sometimes people want the model to walk on their face, mostly it's toe sucking. Sometimes people want to talk to someone who will listen; they'll pay for the session and just chat," she said.

"Fascinating," I said, stroking my chin and nodding my head.

I *had* to go to one of those sessions.

My curiosity was insatiable. Without thinking about it, I volunteered to be a foot model.

Barbie laughed, "I'd love that! Let me see your feet."

I hesitated. My feet were in no shape for licking. They were dry and calloused from running, and the nails were unpainted and uncut.

I peeled my sock off slowly, under the table and showed her what we were working with.

She swallowed and very graciously suggested I "work on them a little" and would revisit the subject with me in a few months.

Barbie had to leave to film her series. She stood up and gave me a hug. Talking to her had been easy. Even though we'd only been together for an hour or so, I felt like we were already friends. I was excited to support and maybe work with her.

"Email me when your feet are ready," she said, waving goodbye on her way out.

I waited until she was out the door and immediately walked my li'l ol' self straight over to the foot aisle at the closest drugstore. With a shopping cart filled to the brim with lotions, antifungal sprays, pumice stones, and a Ped Egg, I beelined to the checkout to begin my new life as a fabulous, rich foot model of Instagram.

I was determined to be a part of one of Barbie's boutiques and I wasn't leaving anything to chance.

GODDAMNIT, THERE'S STILL A LOT OF SHIT LURKING AROUND

While I was trying to get my feet ready for licking, I had another examine-the-garbage-that's-rotting-around-your-heart, hit-you-in-the-motherfucking-gut therapy session.

I'd been avoiding Dr. D'Souza because "I was busy and it was expensive." At least that's what I told my roommates.

To be honest, the "I'm broke" excuse was no longer valid since I'd gotten a new job teaching public speaking. And the only thing I was busy doing was watching *Big Brother* three times a week.

I was avoiding therapy because it was hard.

With a lot of cajoling from Lindsay, I finally scheduled another appointment. The session began like any other: she asked how I was, and then barraged me with a bunch of difficult questions I didn't really want to answer.

"How are things with Ben?" Dr. D'Souza asked pointedly through the computer screen.

Damnit, I knew I shouldn't have told her about him.

"I mean, it's going nowhere. He has no plans to come here and I have no plans to go there," I said.

"Why are you texting him then?" she said.

"I don't know. It's fun? Validation? You're the therapist here," I said, sassier than I needed to be.

"Do you think you're a confident person?" she asked.

Straight for the throat. I guess I deserved that for being such a smart aleck.

"Yeah, for the most part," I said.

"Are you confident in your relationships?"

"With my friends and family, I'd say yes. But romantic relationships? Probably not."

"Why do you think that is?" she asked.

"I don't know," I said.

"Think about it," she encouraged kindly, even though I was being a jerk.

I sat there silently, running through reasons why I wouldn't feel confident in relationships. I started having flashbacks to high school and all the times I'd been rejected subsequently. My eyes started to water but before any tears could fall, I wiped them with a leftover Chipotle napkin.

"I guess . . . when I was younger, no one wanted me. I mean, I was never the girl anyone wanted to date. Like, even in college, we'd go out and everyone would get hit on but me."

"When was the first time you ever felt wanted?"

"I guess when I went to Brazil and fell in love with Gustavo."

Gustavo was my first love. He had broken my heart a dozen tiny times. I was devastated when it ended.

We hadn't been together in over twelve years.

It had been a long and tumultuous healing process that involved two years of not speaking and then a few years of tentative friendship before we could become actual friends.

"What happened?"

We'd been over this before, so I kept it short and simple, "He fell in love with someone else."

"Why?"

I knew she was trying to help me, but I was annoyed. I didn't see how Gustavo was relevant to any of this. It was a long time ago and I was over it.

"I don't know. Why do you fall in or out of love with anyone?" I said irritably.

"How was she different from you?"

"She was thin and beautiful," I snapped.

A silence hung between us.

The gravity of what I'd said and the implications of what it meant about how I felt about myself was too much. I had confessed that I believed that my first love wouldn't have stopped loving me if I was thinner.

This time I couldn't contain the tears. They flowed freely down my face until the Chipotle napkin was soaked.

I needed a few moments to recover, the napkin crumpled in my hand. Dr. D'Souza waited patiently; she didn't offer kind words or try to get me to move on to the next question.

Eventually my sniffling stopped and when I was ready, she asked, "Do you think you're attractive?"

"Sometimes."

"Do you act like you think you're attractive?"

"No."

I wanted to be confident in dating but the truth was that middle school me, the girl who was overweight and unpopular, was still there sometimes. There was a little voice inside of me saying, "He'll leave you for a thinner, prettier gymnast with a perfect body." I was worried that I was going to spend my whole life believing that I wasn't good enough to be with someone.

There was nothing lamer than low self-esteem ruining your life. I needed to do something, but what?

How does someone raise their self-esteem?

We talked about some strategies and by the time we finished the call, I felt shitty.

I perused the self-help section on Amazon and bought a bunch of books that promised to make me into a badass who didn't give a fuck.

For the next few weeks, I listened to motivational videos on YouTube starring Lisa Nichols, Les Brown, and Marisa Peer. I stuck sticky notes on my wall that said, "I am enough." I made a list of things I was grateful for every morning.

In some ways, it worked. I was essentially brainwashing myself to have a more positive response to negative thoughts. I was starting to feel good again.

It wasn't quite sufficient though.

I googled, "How to feel confident while dating."

An article popped up with the headline "Ten Tips to Be a Self-Assured Dater"

It was written by a pickup artist.

Most of it was crap, but some of it made sense.

A lot of sense, actually.

So much sense that later that night I contacted my friend Eric Felter.

SECRETS FROM A TOP PICKUP ARTIST

The mission: rack up rejections.

How?

By hitting on at least five people who I thought were objectively more attractive than me. The more rejections, the better.

Why?

Eric called it "Rejection Immunization." He said that the easiest way to feel more confident was to stop giving so many shits.

To be honest, I gave a lot of shits. It was one of my biggest problems. I really cared what other people thought of me. I wanted to be someone who didn't. Or *at least* someone who could discern when to care and when to not give a shit.

Eric Felter was six-foot-one with a perfect body and a smile that made people (me) melt. He was also a top-rated pickup artist. Number six in the world to be exact.

He won the title at a PUA (Pickup Artist) convention, though *how* exactly he'd won was a mystery to me. Every time I asked him, he skirted the question. I wasn't sure if he was being intentionally vague or if he didn't know either.

Hiring a pickup artist was my latest idea in my quest for coitus. After my last therapy session, I wasn't feeling great about myself.

If anyone could help me feel more confident, it was Eric.

Everything I knew about PUA came from the 2007 MTV show *The Pickup Artist*. The main takeaway was that by using the right techniques, even nerdy men in furry hats could leave with models. I was hesitant to explore the world of PUA because it felt predatory to me.

Eric insisted this wasn't the case. He said that PUA was about communication and getting over the fear of rejection. If that was true, then it was worth a try.

Eric agreed to teach me how to confidently walk in a bar and hit on men, even though he was "retired" from the PUA world. He liked the challenge of working with someone who hadn't had sex in five years.

Plus, we were friends, though I had known him for a whole year before I learned about his past life as a pickup artist.

We met up in the middle of the week at a trendy bar in the Meatpacking District for my first lesson.

He showed up wearing a zip-up hoodie and sneakers. His casual clothes didn't detract from the fact that he was hot. Like ridiculously hot. He was one of the best-looking men I knew, which I assumed helped him pick up women.

"Of course this is easy for *you*. You're super attractive," I said while changing into the heels I had brought for the evening. I hadn't worn heels in weeks because I was still trying to get my feet in shape for Barbie's boutique.

Eric vehemently disagreed that looks were everything. He said he had coached thousands of people. Millionaires, models, and regular ol' people like me.

Good to know that even the plebes like me had a chance.

"The honest to God truth is that it doesn't matter. There's someone out there for everyone. I've worked with attractive people who were insecure, and they struggled far more than clients who might be considered conventionally unattractive," Eric said.

I liked that answer.

There was someone out there for everyone.

Even a celibate.

"Alright, Dr. Phil," I said, smirking. "Let's get to the nitty-gritty. I want some tips and tricks. Like what about peacocking and kino escalation?"* I asked as we walked into a Biergarten with a giant backyard, plenty of picnic tables, and lights strung end to end. They sold boots of beer that had to be purchased with tickets and pretzels the size of a baby's face. It was a popular spot for young male professionals to grab an after-work drink. Tonight was no exception. The place was packed even though it was a Wednesday. Most of the clientele looked about twenty-four. They were wearing suits, but it was just as easy to imagine them in polos at a frat house.

Eric sighed, "Forget everything you think you know about PUA. This isn't about manipulating someone into liking you. Granted, some members of the seduction community might believe in that crap, but it isn't what I'm teaching you."

"What are you teaching me then?" I asked.

"Communication and connection," he said. "We try too hard to make our puzzle piece match someone else's puzzle piece. It's a crapshoot. While you're trying to become who they want, they're busy trying to become who you want. Four dates in, you realize no one is who they were pretending to be. I'm going to teach you how to show up and communicate authentically, exactly as you are."

---

* I had read about these on the Internet. Peacocking was the art of wearing something crazy or some sort of accessory that helped you stand out from the crowd. Kino escalation was about slightly increasing touch to build tension and connection.

The objective for the evening was to reduce my fear of rejection. According to Eric, most people were single because they took rejection personally.

We were going to start with "the open, stay, close" which was just a fancy way of saying that I would initiate conversations by confidently approaching people, finding some common ground to talk about, and if I was interested, giving them my number.

"Okay, what do I do?" I asked.

"Ask these girls where the restroom is," he said.

Too easy. I did that all the time.

As if reading my mind, he gave me a look that said, "We're just getting started."

He was ruthless, forcing me to open conversations in rapid succession.

"Ask these guys where to get your drink tickets."

"Tell this woman her top is nice."

"We're done warming up. Now pick someone you find attractive," he said.

I spotted a Jason Segel look-alike (good-looking yet approachable) by the ping-pong table and decided to hit on him first. My palms were clammy as I approached him.

"How do you sign up for the table?" I asked, trying to look confident and calm.

Open, complete.

He told me, and I transitioned into asking him how often he played and where he learned, which lead to a conversation about his college dorm, which was, ta-da, in my home state of Ohio.

Stay, complete.

We bonded over our love of the greatest state in the union (people from Northeast Ohio are hyper into Ohio), so that gave us a lot to talk about.

"Why don't you take my number? That way you can let me know when the table is open," I said. He smiled devilishly and accepted my offer.

Close, complete.

Oh my God, I had done it.

I had approached a man at a bar and given him my number and it was surprisingly easy. I was a confident, badass mofo. If only Dr. D'Souza could see me now.

I moved toward the bar to find my second target.

"What's the best drink here?" I asked the man next to me. (Open.)

"I only drink whiskey but whatever you get, ask for the free popcorn."

We connected over our love of bar popcorn, which led to a conversation about what movie we had seen most recently, which for both of us was the latest Marvel flick. (Stay.)

I closed by asking for his number.

I had him double-check the number in my phone, walked away, and texted him my name a few minutes later so he'd have it. I received a response almost immediately, "Who?"

I told him we had just met at the bar.

"Wrong number," the message wrote back.

He'd given me a fake number!

I was enraged and told Eric I was going to confront him, but Eric just looked bemused.

"Congrats, my dear, your first rejection of the night! Only four more to go."

"But, c'mon, who does that? I mean seriously, why didn't he just say he had a girlfriend or something?"

"Remember, it's not personal."

It sure felt personal.

If I had been alone, I probably would have called it a night right then and there. I probably would have sulked the whole train ride home, changed into my jammies, and said "fuck it" to dating ever again. Since Eric was doing me a favor by not charging me for the lesson, I didn't want to let him down by giving up that quickly.

I approached someone else and didn't get past the open. He had no interest in talking to me, and after a few tries, I had even less interest in talking to him. Rejection number two or, as Eric called it, "Nexting," which meant disengaging with someone who seemed uninterested.

I moved on. Eric had changed my mind about this being predatory. I showed up to every conversation authentically myself. If there was nothing to talk about and no common ground, then I had to move on. In his words, it wasn't about trying to force a connection with everyone. It was a numbers game, where the more people I talked to, the more likely I was to connect with some of them.

"Learn something about the man behind you in the leather jacket," Eric instructed.

This was the first one I didn't want to do. The man in the leather jacket was an eleven out of ten, probably a model or an actor. I bet he only dated beautiful, tall women with flowing hair and flat stomachs.

I didn't think I could handle three rejections in a row even if that was supposed to be the point.

Seeing my hesitation, Eric said, "The outcome doesn't matter. Remember, it's about reducing your fear of rejection."

"Dude, that guy is out of my league. Don't make me do it," I said.

"No, he isn't. Now go talk to him. What's the worst that can happen?"

"He'll be like 'Why are you talking to me?' Or glare at me like I don't exist, and my face will get so hot that I'll combust into flames becoming the first person ever to *literally die* of embarrassment." I said, throwing my hands up.

He gave me a look that implied, "Are you done yet?"

"Fine," I grumbled.

I turned toward the man, walking fearlessly, before making a sharp left turn and heading toward the bathroom.

I needed a few seconds to rev myself up. I texted Eric from the stall, "Whoops, had to pee!" I checked my Facebook, responded to some emails, and dilly-dallied as long as I could.

I looked at myself in the mirror. "You got this." I reapplied my lipstick, paced the floor a few times, put a piece of gum in my mouth, paced some more, and left to find Eric waiting for me outside.

"You're sexy and fearless. Now go talk to the guy in the leather," he said.

"Yeah! I'm sexy and fearless," I repeated. "I am sexy and fearless," I whispered to myself a few times as I meandered toward him, taking a loop before winding up behind him and his friend.

I stood there, lurking like a total Gollum, knowing I had to say something before he turned around. I tapped him on the shoulder.

"Uh . . . Excuse me. Um. Do you know how to get drink tickets here?"

This was already going less smoothly than my other opens.

He turned around.

"It's over there," he said with a thick accent, pointing toward the ticket counter.

I recognized that accent.

I'd heard that accent many times.

"Are you Brazilian?" I asked in perfect Portuguese.

His face broke into a deep grin. "You speak Portuguese?"

Before long we were laughing and flirting.

I looked over at Eric, and he gave me a thumbs-up and then a sign to indicate that it was time to move on.

I made an excuse to leave, knowing that I had to close. Luckily, he took the lead for me.

"I'm having a cookout tomorrow, you should come," he said.

Be cool. Be cool.

"Yeah, that's sounds fun," I said, putting my number in his phone.

He leaned down to kiss me on my cheek, Brazilian-style.

When I was out of his line of vision, I squealed to Eric, "He took my number!"

"Of course he did. You're delightful," Eric said.

I was feeling good about myself.

If Leather Jacket took my number, I had a chance with anyone.

Now that I had a few wins under my belt, I was unstoppable, I was just a few "opens and closes" away from meeting the love of my life and having the greatest sex ever, which I told Eric, half-jokingly.

"Do you honestly think you're going to find the love of your life at the bar like this?" Eric asked.

"Maybe," I said.

He looked skeptical.

"You're probably not going to meet your lifelong partner at a hookup bar on a Wednesday night in the Meatpacking District. What you are going to do is learn how to reduce your fear of talking to someone, and *then* use those skills when you find someone who makes sense with you. At yoga. Or the library."

"Why do I always gotta be in the library category? Why don't I ever get put in the 'club' category?" I complained.

"Do you go to clubs?"

"No, but I *could.*"

Eric laughed, "Take it as a compliment. Librarians are sexy. You got this whole 'girl next door' vibe going on and you're also funny. It's cool."

Before I could assess whether or not Eric was hitting on me, he gave me my next assignment.

Two men casually drinking by the ping-pong tables: a guy in glasses and a man in plaid.

I approached them and asked where I could get the drink tickets.

"Do you guys come here often?" I asked. It wasn't an original question, but it was a decent conversation-starter.

We chatted for fifteen minutes and Glasses seemed interested in me. I was definitely interested in him. He was clever and quick with a joke.

Everything was going fine until he turned abruptly toward me and said, point-blank, "You knew how to buy drinks here, didn't you?"

So far, no one had called me out.

I was a terrible liar, so I had to come clean.

"I did, but I saw two handsome men and needed an excuse to talk to them."

Holy crap, I had officially become the new Rico Suave.

I could have stopped there, and I would have been charming. An expert PUA. Unfortunately, in true Olive fashion, I overexplained by adding information he hadn't asked for.

"I'm here with a pickup artist and he's teaching me how to hit on men because I'm writing a book about dating," I said.

Glasses laughed but there was no warmth in the laughter.

He didn't believe me.

"Okay, let's say that's true. Where is he then?"

I looked around and couldn't find Eric. He had picked the most inopportune time to go to the bathroom. When I couldn't find him, they thought I was making the whole thing up.

"Let's say you're 'with a pickup artist,' then you're learning how to manipulate people?" Glasses said.

"No, no, no. That's not it at all. I'm trying to not feel intimidated by men I find attractive. How's it going so far?" I said, trying to save the situation.

"You can tell your 'pickup artist friend,' if he exists, that you did just fine," Glasses replied.

Eric returned, and I could see him in my periphery. I expected him to hit on women while he was waiting for me, but he didn't, opting instead to sit at the bar alone, sipping water.

When he saw me look at him, he got up and came over.

"You ready? I've got to go to bed early tonight. Let's get going?"

He walked away.

Glasses shook his head, "Ohhhh, he exists. Good-looking dude. But seriously, you don't need a pickup artist to help you hit on men. I can't understand why you would be having any problem meeting people."

"Thanks," I said, running off to meet Eric, some of my shyness kicking back in.

"Did you close?" Eric asked once we were outside of the bar.

"No, I couldn't tell if he was interested or not."

"Well are you interested enough to get his number or give him yours?"

"Yeah, but I can't go back in," I said.

"Sure you can, I'll wait for you here."

I walked back into the bar slowly, reminding myself that I was brave and rejection didn't faze me.

I walked up to Glasses, and said, "Are you single? Can I have your number?"

"Oh look, she's back! Looking for a story. And no," he said.

I felt a little defensive; that was more aggressive than I had expected.

"I'm not looking for any sort of story," I said.

"No, I'm not single," he clarified.

Now it was awkward, especially because I had already left the bar and come back. I knew I shouldn't have come back in. I couldn't figure out why he had wasted twenty minutes flirting with me if he wasn't single.

There was no graceful way to leave a second time so I just said. "Okay then. Bye."

I rejoined Eric outside and seeing the look on my face he reminded me that it would get easier the more I did it. Getting rejected was good because it made me less sensitive.

By the end of the night I had gotten three rejections and successfully given my number to two people. I wasn't overly excited about any of the successes and I wasn't destroyed by any of the failures. That was progress.

I didn't think I had met the future Mr. Persimmon, but Eric was right, it got easier the more I did it.

"How'd I do?" I asked Eric as we walked toward the subway.

He told me I was a model student and should practice a few more times before saying, "Listen, you don't need me. You're a capable, smart, attractive woman living in NYC. You know how to communicate. If you're not dating, it's because you're not putting yourself out there."

It was the second time I wondered if he was hitting on me.

He was right, though; it was time to start putting myself out there. But how?

BRINGING SEXY BACK

Twenty blind dates in thirty days.

That was my latest and greatest idea for how to "put myself out there" as Eric had suggested. I had been working on the internal crap for months and I wanted to get back into the dating scene for real.

Normal people just downloaded Tinder but I thought it might be more fun to post a status on Facebook asking friends and acquaintances to set me up with their favorite bachelors. To my surprise, the post resulted in twenty blind dates.

I was booked solid for the month. I had dates on Mondays, Tuesdays, and Wednesdays. Dates for breakfast. Dates booked for lunch. I was exhausted just thinking about it. We met at coffee shops and bars. We went on walks and ate dinners. I wore my red top, my black off-the-shoulder dress, and then Febrezed my red top to wear again. For the most part, my friends set me up with thoughtful and kind men. Despite this, most of them were first dates only.

Until Simon.

He was blind date number nine, a setup from a trusted friend, Brian.

We arranged to meet at a park for a picnic on one of the hottest days of the summer. I wiped the sweat off my forehead and hoped he wouldn't notice the glossiness of my face as I reapplied my blush for the second time that day.

I paced around the park entrance waiting for him to arrive when I received a text saying that he thought he saw me.

We had exchanged pictures beforehand but when he approached, I was delighted to see that he was even better-looking in person, five-foot-ten with dark blond, curly hair swooped to one side. His plaid shirt accentuated his lean build. A long scar down the side of his face added a sense of mystery. He was definitely sexy.

"Olive?"

"You must be Simon. Nice to meet you," I said.

We found an old park bench next to a pond and wiped away chipped pieces of paint before sitting down. He had brought a bag of hot dog buns so we could feed the ducks, even though we were sitting next to a large sign that said we weren't supposed to. After getting through the basic small talk, we both relaxed and conversation started to flow easily. He was charismatic and funny.

"So, you're a writer?" he asked, grabbing a hot dog bun and tearing it into small pieces.

"Yep!" I said, feeling cautious about this detail after the reaction from Glasses at the bar.

"That's so cool! I'm a writer myself. Brian mentioned that you're writing a book about sex to 'break your dry spell' and you're exploring all sorts of crazy stuff?"

Talk about laying all the cards on the table. I was relieved that he already knew though, the thought of telling a new prospect about my inexperienced past gave me anxiety.

"Yeah, it's been an interesting year! What do you write about?" I responded.

"It's mostly just a bunch of meandering thoughts, but I want to write more. That's why I was excited for this date. To be honest, this is only the second date I've been on since I've moved to New York." He shared that he had moved from Arizona a few months before and was settling into city life.

"Tell me about your life in Arizona."

"Honestly, a lot of drugs in the desert. I wore vests . . . like macramé vests," he said, simultaneously laughing and rolling his eyes. "The last few years were a little weird. I moved here because I needed a change."

He entertained me with more stories about his life in Arizona and how he had taken a job in NYC walking dogs to pay his rent. The conversation bounced around effortlessly, both of us making jokes.

"Tell me something totally weird about yourself," I said.

"Okay, I've got one. I love to eat rotisserie chicken with my bare hands, ripping it right off the bone," he said with enthusiasm, raising both hands to his mouth, and baring his teeth to recreate the image.

"I love it," I said, laughing.

He shared intimate information about his life with ease and humor. He listened as much as he talked, laughed at my jokes, and asked me questions about my own stories.

The date felt easy, like hanging out with an old friend I had known for years.

An hour in and I wanted to touch him. Badly.

But I still couldn't tell if he liked me. He made no effort to leave but also no effort to be obviously flirtatious. It seemed like we were just two good friends having a nice evening in the park.

We sat on the bench, side by side, for three hours. It was the first date of all my blind dates where I wasn't watching the clock. I hadn't checked my phone and even though it was getting dark, I didn't want it to end.

The park wasn't safe at night, though, so we got up to leave, walking slowly, neither one of us really sure where we were going.

"Do you have to get home soon?" I asked, uncertain if he wanted to keep hanging as much as I did.

"No, do you?" he said.

"Nope. Let's go for a walk." I suggested.

"I'd love that. But I have to do this first. . . ."

He leaned down, his mouth meeting mine. His lips were warm and open. He kissed me slowly and passionately, sliding his tongue into my mouth. I leaned into him, my body responding, moaning softly into his lips.

I had kissed dozens of boys since my dry spell began, but kissing Simon reminded me that I hadn't truly been kissed in that butter-flies-in-your-stomach sort of way in a long time.

I pulled away, grinning.

As we started walking, he reached down and casually grabbed my hand.

We spent the next three hours walking, kissing, and finding other benches to sit on in between kissing and walking. We stopped in a hidden alcove and he leaned over and kissed my bare shoulder. His lips grazing my skin was enough to make me shiver in pleasure.

"This is nice," I said, leaning over to kiss him again.

"Really nice," he said, running his finger over my palm.

We reluctantly ended our date six hours after it began, my face plas-tered with a dopey grin the whole way home. I couldn't remember the last time I'd had a date like that.

I'd had a crush on Adam; I'd kissed Ben. This was different from all of those. It was the best date I had been on in years.

Maybe ever.

On the way home, I touched my lips, trying to remember the feeling of his. I couldn't fall asleep because I wanted to replay the night over and over, trying to burn it into my memory. It was enough fodder for masturbation for days.

He texted me the next morning, "Thoroughly enjoyed myself yesterday. Would love to see you again."

For our second date, we met for coffee. On our third date, I met his friends and his brother. Both times felt magical. This boy was doing weird things to me. My body felt tingly and warm even when he wasn't around.

On our fourth date, we went to the Metropolitan Museum of Art. We took our time, strolling through the rooms, taking long breaks to make out in corners. We couldn't keep our hands off each other. Standing across from a Monet, I looked at his face and smiled happily. He caught me looking at him and smiled back, squeezing my hand.

I was falling for him, hard.

For lunch, we headed to the museum café and cozied up to each other on the bench. He placed his notebook, the one he always carried in his back pocket, on the table. I imagined it was full of poems, brilliant thoughts, and musings from the mind of this wonderful boy. The writer in me appreciated his need to have a paper and pen at any given time.

He saw me eyeing it and said, "It's mostly stupid to-do lists and groceries. Nothing of importance."

"May I?" I asked, curious to see what was on this boy's grocery list. I wanted to know everything about him. Did he buy a lot of rice? What did he eat for breakfast? This was all valuable information if I was ever going to move into girlfriend zone.

"Of course," he said, handing it to me.

I flipped open to a random page and silently read, "For years, I've showered her with affection and love but she gives me nothing in return."

It was dated a week before.

Two days after our third date.

My heart plummeted.

Fuck. Fucccccccck.

Of course. Things were going too well.

He looked over my shoulder to see where I landed and when he saw what I was seeing, an uncomfortable silence rolled over us.

I broke the silence first, "You don't have to tell me. We're new, this is only our fourth date. You don't owe me any explanations," I said, trying to mask my uncertainty about what this new revelation meant.

He was silent for another minute, his face getting visibly emotional. His eyes filled with tears and when he spoke, his voice was shaky.

"That's about . . . it's about . . . umm . . ." He paused.

I bit my lip, letting him take as much time as he needed.

"It's about my ex-wife. I was married, and we have a child." As he was telling the story, the words rushed out so quickly that I could barely hear them. Her name was Sarah. She got pregnant at seventeen and they were married by eighteen. At twenty-five, she met someone else, divorced him, and moved away with their son. He entered a long depression, which was why he had wound up in the desert doing a lot of drugs.

I was trying to conceal the shock on my face.

He finished telling the story and looked defeated. His eyes brimming with tears, his head downturned. I knew that he assumed that I was going to run for the hills, which, honestly, I was considering. It was a lot. The first boy I had liked in ages came with more baggage than I knew how to handle.

I sat there quietly for a few minutes, trying to process everything I had just heard and trying to figure out how and if I fit into this story at all.

I knew what my reaction should have been. I should have kindly finished the conversation while mentally building a barricade around my heart. I should have asked for some time to think about it carefully before making any decisions. I've dated too many men who were broken over other women.

That's what I *should* have done.

That was the exact opposite of what I wanted to do.

He looked so disheartened that I wanted to grab his face and smother it with kisses. I wanted to smooth his hair and rub the scar that ran down his left cheek and say over and over again, "It's okay." I felt my heart open and pour love at this man. I carefully thought about what I wanted to say, taking my time to make sure I said the right thing.

"I'll follow your lead here. I'd like to know whatever you want to tell me about your past. If you want to talk about it, I'd like that because I want to know about you. And if you don't want to talk about it, that's alright too."

We sat for another fifteen minutes as I cautiously asked him questions, both of us struggling to get our emotional state back to some level of neutral. He didn't touch or reach for me, it seemed like he was too deeply buried in his own grief that it didn't matter if I was there or not.

We walked around the museum for another hour. He changed the topic to lighter things, and as promised, I followed his lead.

Two more hours passed, and we managed to return to some place of normalcy, except now I had the burden of knowledge: Simon came with heavy baggage.

Then again, so did I.

I hadn't had sex in five years. I was writing a book about it.

For many people, those would be deal breakers.

They hadn't been for Simon. He showed up to our first date anyway.

We left the museum to grab dinner downtown but before we did, he kissed me with great care and intensity on the front steps of the museum. In that kiss was everything we had left unsaid.

On his end it said, "Thank you for listening. I'm glad you're still here and yes, I am sad." On my end it said, "I'm still here, everyone has a past."

We went downtown and shared dinner and despite the revelations from earlier in the day, I still felt happy.

We moved from dinner to a bookstore. From the bookstore to a stroll. From the stroll to a bench where we made out like teenagers.

The date lasted twelve hours and by the end of it, I still wasn't tired of him.

He left for vacation the next day which gave me some much-needed time to reflect.

I lay in my bed that night and reviewed the facts:

Simon had an ex-wife.
He had a son.
He was divorced.
That was six years ago.
He was still sad about his divorce.

While he was gone, I analyzed the entire situation with intense unease. If overthinking was an Olympic sport, I would have won three gold medals that week alone.

I thought about him. And me. And what it all meant, if it meant anything.

While I was busy thinking and worrying, there was one feeling that was stronger than all of the others.

I missed him.

I wanted to see him and kiss him and continue dating him.

He came back from vacation and met me one night in the park in a crisp blue button-down shirt that highlighted his new golden tan. He wasn't just good-looking, he was straight out of a *GQ* magazine. I couldn't focus on anyone else. We sat down and made out until I noticed a poetry reading going on across the park.

"Want to watch the reading?" I asked.

"No, I want to watch you." He said, brushing a strand of hair away from my face and leaning in to kiss me. "I'm perfectly content sitting here and kissing you."

In that exact moment I decided to have sex with him. Maybe it was the way he touched my face. Maybe it was the way he was brushing his lips across mine. Maybe there was some magic in the air that only happens late at night when the city is lit up and the windows look like fireflies.

With his arm wrapped around me, we discussed all the heavy topics like God, politics, and whether the correct terminology was "pop" or "soda." We talked about why we loved and hated NYC before moving on to our morning coffee routines.

"I drink shitty coffee. I buy it at this weird deli by my house, it smells like cats. The deli I mean, not the coffee. It's one dollar for the world's shittiest coffee." he said.

"I use a French press," I said. "We still buy cheap coffee from a can, but we make it in a French press, so it *feels* fancy."

"I haven't had French-pressed coffee since I lived in Arizona," he said, stroking my hand.

Without giving myself the opportunity to overthink, I paused, before meeting his gaze. "Would you like to have some tomorrow morning?"

He examined my face carefully. "Are you inviting me over?"

"I am," I said.

"Are you sure?"

"I am."

He leaned in and kissed me with a kiss full of promise, his tongue nudging and gently circling mine.

We took our time getting home. Simon and I were classic oversharers so there was no mystery about what was going to happen. We talked about everything and covered the basics of having sex and discussed how we liked to cuddle.

Unfortunately, by the time we got to my apartment, I was starting to panic.

He had never been to my house before.

We had never seen each other naked.

Now we were gonna do the thing that I hadn't done in five years and my cortisol was firing in excess.

I wasn't sure what the next step was, so I grabbed his hand and led him down the hall toward my room.

When we got there, I pulled off my shirt self-consciously, sucking in my stomach while simultaneously trying to look relaxed.

He took his shirt off, pausing to say, "I should have told you, I haven't done this in over a year . . . I'm a little rusty."

Tell me about it. The insecurity radiating off of both sides was palpable.

We crawled into my twin bed.

He kissed me without the ease we normally had.

What happened after that was a blur. There was some sort of exchange of oral pleasantries, but we didn't fool around for too long. We were both too in need of penetrative sex.

I grabbed a condom and opened it, handing it to him to put on.

"Are you sure?" he asked.

I nodded, "Yes. Be gentle, it's been a while."

"Of course."

He leaned down and kissed me. A man of his word, he entered gently.

I flinched.

"Are you OK?" he asked.

"It hurts a little, but don't stop," I said. I wanted to enjoy it, but my brain was racing. I liked him so much and I wanted this to be good, but I couldn't be fully present because I was too in my head about all of it.

We weren't engulfed in the throes of passion, but we were doing this. He was slow and steady, checking in often to make sure I was all right. We continued this way for what seemed like forever until he increased the pace and force.

His moaning intensified until he finally collapsed on top of me.

We lay there for a long time, him still inside of me, not speaking before he got up slowly, pulled off the condom, threw it away, and climbed back in bed.

I rolled away from him. We didn't touch or talk, both stewing in our thoughts. We'd just had bad sex and it was all my fault because I couldn't relax.

I was certain this was the end.

I fell asleep, briefly, negative thoughts in my head. I woke up a half hour later and rolled over to find him still awake.

I was grateful for the darkness in my room and finally worked up the nerve to say, "I'm kind of in my head right now."

"Me too. It's been a long time for me as well."

Silence fell over us again, which was deeply uncomfortable for two people who loved to talk.

"What are you thinking?" he asked.

I knew I could lie, but I didn't see what good lying was going to do if our relationship was on the verge of being over anyway.

"I'm worried that . . . because I haven't had sex in forever that it was bad. Like I've been out of the game for too long and I don't remember how to do it."

He rolled over to face me and reached for my face.

"No, no, no, baby. That's not it," he said softly. "Sex isn't about being 'good' or 'bad.' It's not about mechanics. It's about the connection you have with that person. That's what makes any sex good or bad. Your body takes care of the rest."

I nodded. I wasn't sure I believed him.

"I'm crazy about you. We did this all wrong," he said, shaking his head.

He leaned in and kissed me tenderly and with that kiss my insecurity melted away.

I kissed him back, increasing the intensity as he moved from my face to my neck.

He kissed his way down my neck.

He stopped to lick my collarbone, sucking on it as he worked his way down.

He moved toward my breast and gently flicked his tongue across my nipple. Teasing it, taking his time.

"This is what I should have done," he said.

Perhaps because we were tired or because our brains had just released a surplus of feel-good hormones, we were both more relaxed.

He ran his hands down my stomach, his mouth trailing behind.

This time when he entered me I was ready to go and the pain, while still mildly there, was significantly less.

This time we rocked in sync, both of us moaning, until finally I said, "I'm going to cum."

He came a few minutes later and we laid there entangled, breathing heavily, aimlessly groping for each other, intertwining our bodies, kissing and trying to get closer before we both fell asleep.

When we woke up, we had sex again in the morning.

Unfortunately, the insecurity was back, and it felt more like the first time than the second time.

We didn't have time for coffee because he had to get to work. He left quickly and kissed me on his way out the door.

I sat down on my couch and wrapped a blanket around me.

Holy crap, I did it, I thought.

I had actually broken the dry spell. Five years of celibacy and I *finally* had sex with someone I really, really liked.

I had been waiting for this moment for a long time. It was a big deal to me. I should have been dancing on clouds, but I wasn't.

I was too busy doing math.

One round of awkward sex.

One round of intimate, passionate sex.

And one round of just-okay, average sex.

I wasn't great at math, but those odds didn't seem to be in my favor.

Despite Simon's earlier assurances that sex was about connection, I was worried.

What if he didn't like me anymore? What if we didn't have chemistry? What if our average sex reminded him that he wanted to get back together with his ex-wife? Had I blown any chance I had at being in a relationship or having sex again? Was I destined to be single for the rest of my life?

The questions and worries started to consume me and in about ten minutes I started having a full-on panic attack. I sat on my couch, crying heavily until I couldn't breathe. I was positive he was going to end things with me and tell all his friends that I was an awkward lover.

I called Lindsay until she finally talked me off the ledge. "You're jumping to a lot of conclusions here. Why don't you just call him?"

"I can't do that!" I protested.

A few hours passed and the more I thought about it, the more I realized I actually could do that.

I took a few deep breaths, put on a fake smile to try to convince myself that I wasn't nervous, and called Simon.

He answered on the first ring.

"Hey!" he said.

"Hey you. I'm just calling to, you know, see how you are and make sure you're not too in your head."

"I'm good." I could tell he was smiling from his tone. "Are you in your head?"

"Absolutely."

We both laughed and then talked for another hour.

By the time we hung up, my worries were gone.

Our next date was a day at the beach. Another twelve-hour date by the time it was done.

We headed back to his house and when we got home we showered together, making love as the water dripped down our bodies.

We had sex two times that night, and again in the morning.

When I woke up the next day he was making French toast and potatoes, classical music playing in the background. I wrapped my arms around him while he was cooking, and we swayed together happily.

"Good morning, gorgeous," he said, pausing to kiss me.

"Good morning, sexy," I said.

We ate lazily, breaking to take syrupy kisses.

As we sat holding hands, I wondered if this is what it felt like to belong with someone.

We stopped in his deli for shitty dollar coffee. He was right; it did smell like cats.

As he walked me to the train, I couldn't stop smiling. For the first time in my life, I was maybe, possibly someone's girlfriend.

FOOT WORSHIP, IT'S A THING.
YOU SHOULD TRY IT.

Nine times.

That's how many times Simon and I'd had sex so far. I knew it wasn't normal to count but when the number was as low as mine, it was hard not to. I was afraid it was all a dream. I'd wake up one day and still be an active member of the celibate circus.

We still hadn't defined the relationship, but I knew he wasn't seeing anyone else.

The more comfortable we got with each other, the more we explored. Even though I hadn't quite conquered the basics, I wanted to make up for lost time and figure out what to try with Simon. After all, I'd had five years to think about sex and now that I was finally having it again, I wanted to try everything.

Or close to everything.

Or at least just master reverse cowgirl for crying out loud. (We *still* hadn't done it.)

I also wanted to try some of the kinkier stuff, but I wasn't sure what.

I remembered my conversation with Barbie. Over a million people watched videos of her feet. That number was too high to ignore. People *loved* feet.

But *why*?

Although I was fascinated by it, I still wasn't convinced that feet were going to be a part of my sexual awakening. Feet were gross. End of story. At least that's how I felt until I tried it for myself.

On a feisty evening, I kissed my way down Simon's calf.

I stopped by his ankle and examined his foot. It looked clean and smooth, lightly calloused but definitely not disgusting.

I held his foot with both hands, massaged it, pressing my thumb against the arches, alternating with light touches and strokes from my fingers. I moved to his toes and massaged each one individually, applying pressure the way I liked when I received a massage.

I leaned forward, tentatively, and with some hesitation. I licked my lip and then ran my tongue across his sole. It tasted like skin, as if I had licked his arm. I had heard rumors of a distinctive foot taste, but I didn't notice anything out of the ordinary.

To my surprise, he cried out in pleasure.

I looked at him and raised my eyebrows.

"Oh yeah?"

He nodded, surprised himself.

"I've never done this before," I cautioned.

"Me either but that felt amazing," he said.

That was all I needed. I grabbed his large toe in my mouth, sucking it slowly. His body responded convulsively with whimpers and moans. I ran my tongue between his toes and grabbed for his erection.

I wasn't thinking about the taste or smell of his feet. The only thing I could think about was watching his body twist with pleasure. It made me feel powerful that I was capable of causing that response so easily. I took my time nibbling his ankle, suckling his toes, and watching his body go crazy. Each moan emboldened me to explore even more.

The next time, a few days later, I didn't hesitate or offer an explanation; I grabbed his foot and aggressively sucked on his toes, soaking them in my saliva. I nibbled the sole, flicked my tongue across his heel, and massaged his legs. There was a slight "foot taste" this time but it wasn't bad or distracting.

Once again, I watched his body twist.

This wasn't about curiosity anymore. I had become a goddamned convert. I was a Sole Sorceress, a Toe Tease, a Foot Femme Fatale. I was excited that inexperienced me had discovered a new way to make his body tremble with something he hadn't tried before.

While I was busy licking Simon's feet, I was still trying to convince Barbie to let me be one of her foot models. I wanted to see what it was like to have my own foot worshipped and licked by a stranger. I had made considerable progress in the last few months and spent practically half of my life's fortunes trying to get my feet in order.

I emailed Barbie pictures to convince her to let me be one of her models. To my surprise, Simon said he was okay with all of it. After all, he knew I was writing a book when he started dating me. Two weeks passed with no word from Bar, even though my feet were ready to go.

By the time I heard back from her, Simon changed his mind. He told me he'd been thinking about it and he actually wasn't cool with some random dude licking my foot, even if it was for research.

I understood that, so I told Barbie I'd changed my mind and decided I wasn't interested in modeling.

I continued to investigate on my own. I wasn't aroused by videos or pictures of feet. I didn't incorporate it into the porn I watched but I most certainly incorporated it into my life.

I gave my first foot job to Simon one night when I was feeling particularly lazy. I didn't want to have sex or strain my jaw, so I wrapped my feet around his cock and moved up and down. He watched me with intrigue and excitement. I watched his body contort with pleasure. It was the easiest orgasm I have ever given, a trick for tired women everywhere.

After my repeated successes, I finally understood why feet were a thing. Now I wondered what else was out there.

AN ITCH TO SCRATCH

My friend Ryan was one of my best resources for new, erotic things. He was self-admittedly deep in the fetish scene in NYC. He'd send me articles or connect me to friends of his who were doing cool sex-positive stuff. He kept me in the loop about the sexy comings and goings.

"Ryan! Possibly TMI but I've been exploring foot stuff and I'm curious if there's anything else you might know about," I messaged to him.

"Girl, you know I've got you," he wrote back.

We met up a few days later at a chain falafel joint in Lower East Side.

I sat down on a bench across from Ryan and admired his goofy T-shirt featuring nineties babelicious icon Mario Lopez. Ryan was a comedian, so his wardrobe matched his sense of humor. Usually he was easygoing and quick with a joke but today he looked apprehensive, anxiously chewing his straw.

"Sooo . . . what's up?" I said, pouring some hot sauce on my hummus.

"Well, I wanted to tell you about some, you know, sexy stuff," Ryan said.

"Cool! What is it?"

"Well . . ."

I raised my eyebrows, waiting for him to say something. "I love tickling," Ryan blurted out.

"Huh? Whatchu mean?" I said, shoving a falafel in my mouth.

"I have a tickling fetish. That's the 'something else' you might want to try."

I had been trying to predict what Ryan was going to suggest for days and tickling hadn't even been in the ballpark of what I would have guessed. It wasn't even in the parking lot or on the same street.

"Tell me more," I said. I had never heard of a tickling fetish or even imagined that was a thing.

He was still chewing his straw so I tried to smile to ease his fear.

"Not a lot of people know about this one, so, um, keep an open mind."

"Bro, we're friends and I love you. It's totally cool," I said, grabbing his hand.

He started talking quickly, "I remember the *exact* day I discovered it. My parents were gone, and I typed 'tickling' into the search engine. I remember looking around to make sure no one would catch me. That could have been an innocent thing to search for, but for me, it wasn't."

I put down my fork and leaned forward. I was trying to understand what he was telling me because this was a huge part of his life that I knew nothing about but also because he seemed embarrassed.

"Wait, hold up. You're talking about just tickling right? Like wiggly wiggly," I reached up to imitate a tickling gesture in my armpit.

"Yeah."

"But like sexually?" I said.

"Yeah, it arouses me," he said.

I didn't miss a beat. "Cool!" I said. "You're always surprising me, you with your damn Mario Lopez T-shirt. Want my pickles?" I said with a grin.

He relaxed and finally took the straw out of his mouth, leaning over to scoop them up.

"Now, go on," I encouraged.

"There are two roles. Ticklees and Ticklers. Or Lees and Lers. People who liked to be tickled are Lees; people who do the tickling are Lers."

"Which one are you?" I asked.

"Both, but typically a Lee."

"So you prefer to be tickled?" I asked.

"Yep!"

I thought about which one I would be. Definitely the Ler, with the whole needing to be in control thing and all.

Ryan confessed that he wasn't "out" about this particular fetish. He had only told two of his ex-girlfriends, one was into it and the other one said it "was super weird" and refused to acknowledge it, which explained his initial apprehension in telling me. I was honored that he trusted me.

He found most of his tickling partners online in fetish forums. He didn't have a ton of options because the forum was heavily skewed with men.

With the absence of many willing partners, Ryan occasionally hired women to tickle him.

"Wait, wait, you pay people to tickle you?"

"I mean, yeah, usually other people with a tickling fetish. We meet at hotels and don't have sex or anything. We don't even get fully naked," he said.

"You tickle over your clothes?"

"Yep. Fully-dressed tickling," he said.

"No one gets off? You meet up, tickle each other senseless, and then everyone leaves?"

"Pretty much."

He was being a good sport about answering my questions.

"Fascinating," I said with wholehearted sincerity. I was thrilled to learn that this fetish existed. It was proof that there was still a ton of stuff out there for me to discover.

"If it's just tickling, why the hotels?" I asked.

"Would you want your roommates to walk in on you non-stop laughing for thirty minutes?" he said.

Touché.

"If you ever want to try it, we could have a tickling session," Ryan offered at the end of our meal.

I politely declined. There was no way in hell Simon would be okay with that given his total one-eighty about me trying foot modeling.

Later that night, I called Simon and told him about my lunch and casually mentioned that Ryan had offered to do a session with me.

"You should definitely try it. It's a great story," Simon said.

"What? Are you sure you'd be comfortable with that?"

"It's just tickling, right?" he asked.

"Yeah, that's it," I assured.

"And you and this guy are totally platonic?"

"Absolutely," I said.

"Then you should try it; it's a cool opportunity."

I definitely did not see that coming, but one of my favorite things about Simon was that his curiosity was almost as insatiable as mine.

Four days later, Ryan was standing in my room pulling out his bag of weaponry. Weaponry was the term for the tools used for tickling. His bag included hairbrushes, feathers, and toothbrushes.

I was surprisingly relaxed. There was an easiness to my friendship with Ryan that made me feel comfortable. We approached it like he was giving me an insider's seminar on Tickling 101.

I was going to be the Ler for the first round, which meant Ryan was going to be tickled first. I was happy that I could do this for him and that he didn't have to pay someone.

He went over the weapons and the basic protocol. He advised me to use my fingers first to explore which areas of the body were sensitive. I'd start at the feet and move upward toward the knees. After that I'd tickle the stomach, armpits, inner thighs, and the collarbone. Once I mastered the light touch, I'd experiment with weapons.

While I was examining the weapons, Ryan stripped down to his boxers and laid down on the bed.

I was taken aback; I'd expected this to be a fully clothed session. My mind immediately went to Simon. Even though he knew about the lesson, I wondered if he'd be upset if he knew there was a half-naked man getting tickled in my bed.

If it had been anyone else I probably would have said something.

It's just tickling, I thought, pushing Simon out of my mind.

But was it? I wasn't sure. Perhaps it was naive of me to think it was wholly platonic.

At Ryan's request, I blindfolded and handcuffed him to prevent any involuntary elbowing if the tickling got too intense.

I grazed his foot, gently running my fingers across the soles. Ryan squirmed, and while I thought he might be trying to escape his face was unmistakably happy. Joyous even.

I moved to the back of his knees. No response, so I mentally crossed that off the list of places he enjoyed.

I inched toward his belly and spider-fingered my hand across his stomach. My movement was met with an outburst of squealing laughter. It wasn't a chuckle or a snicker, it was a full-on chortle.

Emboldened by his response, I prematurely grabbed a toothbrush and rubbed the bristles across his armpits and collarbone. With every movement of the brush, Ryan's body responded. He twisted and turned to the stroking, laughing helplessly the entire time.

I laughed too. Partially, because the whole thing was unusual but also in part because it was fun. It was joyful to watch another human being shake with infectious laughter.

Within three minutes we were both roaring loudly. I was laughing so hard that I couldn't breathe.

I noticed that Ryan was slightly erect and thought of Simon again. I suggested he put on pants and we continue with me as the Lee this time.

"Do you want the blindfold?" he asked as he handcuffed me.

"Hell no," I said. Not being able to see was a control freak's worst nightmare. Being handcuffed, which was necessary to prevent elbowing, was already a huge push for me.

I lay down fully clothed on my bed and waited. I hadn't been tickled in years, so I had no idea how this was going to go.

Ryan tickled my feet. No reaction. All my weird chemical foot creams had probably temporarily desensitized them.

He moved from my knees to my belly.

Nothing on either. No reaction or movement on my end.

I was disappointed. Perhaps I just wasn't ticklish anymore. Maybe it was something I had grown out of.

He snaked his way up to my armpit. An outburst of giggles escaped from my mouth.

Jackpot.

I laughed until I was out of breath.

He stopped for a minute to give me a break and moved to my collarbone, this time using the toothbrush.

The bristles grazed my skin and I erupted into a fit of laughter again. Every time I laughed, he laughed. I was surprised by how much I was enjoying myself. Ryan was masterful at the pacing, bringing me right to the edge of painful laughter before releasing me back to normalcy and then back to the brink again.

I was loving it.

I had no idea if, for Ryan, this was erotic and arousing. Maybe his mind was wandering to sweaty, naked places.

For me, it was lighthearted and jolly without being overtly sexual. Perhaps because I was only interested in Ryan as a friend.

Ryan finished tickling me and we both stood in my room, exhausted and sweaty.

Our faces were plastered with grins.

"Thanks for sharing that with me," I said, smiling at him.

"No, thank you!" he said. "It's hard to find someone willing to tickle with me."

I could tell that it was important to him, that it was a part of his identity, a part that was often hidden and unfulfilled.

"Don't pay someone. I'll tickle with you again if you want," I said.

"Thank you," he said sincerely.

"Do you mind if I write about this?"

"Not at all! Just change my name," he said.

Easy enough.

When I started out, I thought fetishes were a weird subset of sex that most of the population couldn't relate to. I lumped all fetishes and kinks together. I thought that people who had them were unrelatable non-conformists who lived on the fringes. Whoever they were, they weren't like me. I was wrong. In fact, like most things I had learned so far, I had no fucking idea what I was talking about.

There were hundreds of fetishes and kinks. The people who had them were bankers and students. Comedians like Ryan. Writers and artists like me. Accountants. People who shopped at Target, responsibly filed their taxes, and raised respectful children.

And yet, Ryan didn't want anyone to know that laughing and tickling turned him on. In some ways it was reassuring. I *knew* that I was sexually repressed, but so was society at large.

I didn't know what to explore next but the realization that I might be into some of the kinkier stuff opened a whole slew of doors that had previously been closed.

I pondered what it would be like to try tickling with Simon. Maybe not as the main event, but definitely as a fun lead-in to playful sex.

I made a mental note that it was definitely something we were going to try.

APPLES AND ORANGES

All the pieces in my life were finally coming together. I had my own room, a job with health insurance, and I was dating a smart man who cooked me French toast.

And finally, *for the love of God finally*, the curse upon my vagina had been lifted.

Simon and I had been dating for a little less than three months. It wasn't long for most people, but it was an eternity for me.

It was everything I wanted. Everything I had asked for, and yet, I couldn't suppress a tiny, nagging feeling that somehow it was all wrong.

My instincts were right, since a few weeks later Simon started acting odd.

Something was up.

He still hadn't officially called me his girlfriend and his communication had become unreliable. Our daily texts became every-other-day texts and he hadn't initiated plans in a while (not that he was ever good at planning). I had no idea when I was going to see him and that frustrated me. The worst part was that we stopped being as physical. He was too tired or not in the mood.

Reverse cowgirl felt like a distant dream.

When we were together we had a great time. The moment he was gone, I felt anxious and afraid that it might be the last time I'd see him. I'd get all worked up and then try to convince myself that I was overanalyzing everything because I hadn't ever been in a real relationship.*

I was constantly evaluating the status of things by checking neat little boxes in my mind. If I made him laugh during a phone call, I'd place a mental check in the "Things Are Fine, You're Thinking Too Much" box. If he didn't text me for a few days, I'd place a check in the "He's Over It" box.

We hadn't been dating very long, but the short honeymoon was over.

"Hey! What are you doing this weekend?" I texted even though I had promised myself that I wasn't going to initiate plans. I hit send with a certain amount of self-loathing for breaking my promise.

He invited me over to his house and offered me leftovers.

He was distant but hospitable.

He was also sick. Simon had been sick for the majority of our relationship. He always had some sort of cold, virus, or sinus infection.

We got into bed and had lazy and unsatisfying sex. When we were done, a breeze blew in through the window. He got up to put a shirt on and so did I.

"Damnit. My tooth hurts," he said, sitting on the edge of the bed, rubbing his cheek.

He had been complaining for weeks about how much his tooth hurt.

"You should make a dentist appointment," I suggested, putting my pants back on.

"I can take care of myself," he snapped, standing up and walking over to grab a bottle of aspirin.

It was the first time he had snapped at me.

---

* The jury is still out on if my Brazilian first love counts as a relationship since 97 percent of it was done long distance.

He wasn't done yet, though. "I've had a long line of women telling me what to do and the last thing I need is another one. Obviously, I have never listened," he said gritting his teeth.

His tone was sharp, and his message was clear: he didn't want me taking care of him. He could take care of himself.

Except he was doing a terrible job at that. He was sick, sad, and broke. He was depressed and anxious. He couldn't or wouldn't prioritize his health.

I didn't know how to deal with anger so I excused myself and cried in the bathroom. I thought he might come after me, but he didn't. When I was done, I crawled back into his bed, where he was already asleep.

When I woke up the next morning he wasn't there. I walked in the kitchen and saw him sitting at the table with scrambled eggs and a glass of Jack, even though it was only 10:30 a.m.

I looked at the whiskey.

"It's for my tooth. I made you an omelet, it's on the stove," he said.

I grabbed my breakfast and sat down, quietly pushing my eggs around my plate, trying not to cry all over again.

"Sorry for being such a jerk," he said, before I could say anything.

"It's fine," I said, blowing it off.

It wasn't fine, though. I was worried about his health. I was worried about us.

He blamed his anxiety on anything and everything: his lack of stable employment, his move to NYC, being alone too much, and a whole host of other things. From my perspective, it seemed like his anxiety came from his divorce. He punished himself by not allowing anyone to care about him. But I wasn't a psychologist, so I didn't say that.

We left his place and walked to the deli to grab coffee.

"Are we okay?" he asked, glancing at me sideways.

"We're okay." I said, grabbing his hand and giving it a squeeze.

I saw Simon the next day and everything felt normal. We laughed, kissed, and made love like nothing had happened at all.

I left for a wedding in Ohio a few days after that and even though things had been normal the last time I had seen him, I was still rattled from our fight.

I didn't want to seem needy so I resolved not to contact him and let him contact me.

Four days in to my trip and I hadn't heard a peep. No calls. No texts. Not even a "like" on Facebook. I wanted him to miss me, but the absence of communication made it seem clear that he didn't, at least not at the level I wanted. I checked my phone every five minutes. I checked to make sure I hadn't accidentally blocked him. I made my friends text me to make sure my phone wasn't broken. The reality was: Simon hadn't/didn't want to contact me.

On day five he sent me a link to a song called "Emotions and Math." I listened to the lyrics and felt reassured.

On day five he sent me a link to a song about a man missing a woman and how he was counting down till she got back.

Oh, he *did* miss me.

I sent him three heart emojis and told him how perfect the lyrics were.

"Oh, I didn't really listen to the lyrics. Just thought you'd like her voice," he wrote back.

My heart dropped.

Seriously? Could he be *that* oblivious?

"The lyrics are about someone being away and someone else missing them."

"Oh. I didn't really think about it."

I sat cross-legged in my childhood bedroom and stewed, feeling foolish for believing there was some sort of hidden meaning in a song, or that he even cared enough to send me something emotionally vulnerable. I didn't respond to his text and went to bed, worrying and thinking. Thinking and worrying.

Somehow it was all wrong.

He didn't text me for the rest of my trip.

I got back on Monday and texted him and he responded with curt replies and no plans to see me. I suggested we meet up on Thursday and advised him to call when he knew his schedule, which, of course, he didn't.

Thursday came, and I was glued to my phone, waiting for him to text. I could have contacted him, but I had too much pride.

His radio silence, also known as ghosting, made it clear that he was trying to end things.

We hadn't dated very long but, goddamnit, we were adults and I deserved better than that. It was cowardly. I wasn't going to quietly fade into the background while he self-destructed and refused to acknowledge my existence in his life. We had been intimate, both emotionally and physically, so the least he could do was muster up some motherfucking courage to actually break up.

"We need to talk," I texted him the next day.

He responded immediately, "Are you free tomorrow?"

We met at the farmers' market by the park. He didn't kiss or hug me, which I was both upset and not upset about. I still thought that maybe, just maybe, this was fixable. We could make this work.

With more communication, I'd feel less anxious. Maybe he'd get a better job and feel more confident. Maybe I could talk to my therapist again. If we could fix all these other variables, then we could make our relationship work.

My brain was running through all the scenarios, though in the burrows of my intuition, I knew that there was only one variable that mattered. He was emotionally unavailable and that made us incompatible. Nothing was going to change that. He was an apple. I was an orange. We made a nice fruit basket but not a great pie.

We sat on a park bench and talked about a bunch of benign topics like the weather and the forages of the farmer's market, both of us too cowardly to start the breakup. It was par for the course, we had spent the majority of our relationship on park benches, bantering about nothing and not saying what we needed to say.

After an hour, I couldn't believe we were still pretending like we didn't know exactly why we were there.

"C'mon, Simon. We need to talk about what's going here," I said, making a gesture toward both of us.

He looked uncomfortable and emotional.

He didn't make any excuses for his behavior and said, "I can't be in a relationship. Obviously, I'm too unstable and my life is too much of a mess to be with anyone right now."

I wanted to tell him that wasn't true, but he was right: his life was a bit messy at the moment.

Even though he was breaking up with me, I was more worried about him than myself.

I had a lot of friends and a strong social circle. After six years in NYC, I was settled. I knew the bars I'd go to drink to forget him. I knew the men I could make out with to rebound. I'd land on my feet. Simon was still relatively new to NYC. I was afraid that he was going to sit around and drink himself into oblivion, that his health was going to get even worse.

We talked, and then talked some more, but I didn't try to convince him to stay. I learned a long time ago that you can't convince someone to stay if they want to go. I could wear my sexiest dress and tell my funniest jokes but no matter what, I couldn't force Simon, or anyone, to love me.

Beneath the surface-level disappointment, I was relieved. In my gut, I knew he wasn't my forever person. He was giving me an out before we became too entangled in each other's lives. I had taken on the burden of making him happy and he was absolving me of that responsibility.

I was grateful for that because, ultimately, you can't make sad people happy. They will only make you sad too.

Though, of course, I couldn't explore that emotion at that exact moment while watching the first man I'd had sex with in five years tell me he didn't want to be with me.

We said our final goodbyes and I got up, waiting to cry until I was out of sight.

I thought about going to the bar, even though it was only 1:00 p.m. I headed toward the bar but couldn't hold it together long enough to get there, so I sat down on a stranger's front stoop and cried until my well was empty.

I cried for our first date, the only date that had made me excited in years. I cried for our fourth date when we spent twelve hours together and our ninth date when I stopped counting how many dates we had gone on. I cried because there were things I was never going to learn about Simon, like how he got the scar on his face or what kind of gloves he wore in the winter. And, truthfully, I cried because I wanted to have more sex. I was just beginning to figure things out.

Strangers walked by and averted their gaze while I sobbed unapologetically in public.

When I was done crying, I got up and did the only think I could think of.

I went home.

A few weeks passed, and I kept hoping that he'd show up with flowers and a card that said, "I messed up." But I knew, deep down, that was never going to happen. He wasn't going to reach out because he meant what he said, he didn't want to be in a relationship with me.

I went on a few dates to occupy my mind, but I kept comparing them to Simon, and when they all fell short, I stopped dating all together.

I needed time to grieve.

Just like that, I had found coitus.

And just like that, my love life stalled again.

THE STUPID THINGS YOU DO
AFTER A BREAKUP

I spent the next few weeks going out A LOT.

I had plans from the moment I woke up until I collapsed into bed. If I was busy, then I was distracted. If I was distracted, then I wasn't thinking about Simon. I slept in late, cried in bathrooms at bars, and drank too much. I ate cold fries and ice cream for breakfast, not once but twice. The guy at my local Taco Bell knew my name, and I didn't even like Taco Bell. I had become a living, breathing twenty-two-year-old break up cliché. Except I was thirty and I probably should have been managing this better.

Given how things were going, it wasn't a surprise that I wound up at the Private Detective Gentleman's Club on a Monday night.

Actually, it *was* a surprise. I hated strip clubs. The first and only time I had been to one was eight years prior in Ohio. A stripper named Destiny clapped her ass in my face while I anxiously put a dollar bill in her G-string. I found a pubic hair in my salad, though in all fairness, it was my fault for ordering a salad at a strip club.

I wasn't a fan.

Unfortunately, *that's* where I was at in life. Needless to say, I wasn't handling my new singleness with grace and ease.

For the record, going to the strip club wasn't my idea.

I was out for a friend's birthday, which started innocently enough with dinner and drinks. Around 10:00 p.m. the couples headed home to have sex and be happy. At least that's what I imagined. Around 11:30 the responsible employed people headed home so they weren't tired for work. I should have been in this category but as a recent dumpee, I was feeling self-destructive and didn't care if I was tired for work. That's what coffee was for.

Even the birthday boy left eventually, leaving four of us behind: Me; Katie, an acquaintance I only saw at events hosted by our mutual friend; and two single men, Kyle and Brendan.

The Single Suckers.

Actually, Katie wasn't single; she was in a long-distance relationship. That left me as the only single female.

I had my eye on Kyle even though he wasn't my normal type. He looked a little too perfect. He had nicer brows than I did and the kind of square jawline that I thought only existed in old-school Disney movies. His skin, body, and outfit were all flawless. We had nothing in common, but I still wanted to make out with him, just to prove to myself that men still wanted me. A make out session with a hottie like Kyle would have been a major ego boost.

We drank at the bar until Katie suggested we go to the gentleman's club.

Apparently, they had a "wing special" that started at 2 a.m.

If Katie hadn't been in a relationship I probably would have called her bluff, but instead I agreed that cheap wings *did* sound like the practical next step.

With twenty-five-cent teriyaki on our minds, or my mind at least, we loaded into a cab and headed uptown to meet our fate.

The gentleman's club was located unapologetically in the middle of a busy street by Times Square. The outside was discreet enough but still boasted posters of scantily clad, beautiful women.

A large, brooding man with a ponytail stood at the front doors, checking IDs.

The entrance was dark with a string of white Christmas lights running around the hostess stand. A young woman in her mid-twenties with impeccably straight hair and leather booty shorts greeted us as we entered.

Or greeted Kyle, I should say.

She immediately zoned in on him, and I wasn't sure if it was because he was handsome or because he looked like he had money.

"Are you looking for a table, sweetheart?" she said, batting her eyelashes at him and touching his shoulder.

"Four, please," he said, flashing her an expensive Disney smile with the type of perfectly straight, white teeth that didn't happen naturally. The hostess grabbed his hand and led him to a table in the middle of a large room. There was a stage in the center with a woman dancing in a neon green, sequin-covered costume and five-inch heels. The perimeter was lined with benches where two men were receiving lap dances.

"Um, can we get the wing menu too, please?" I asked the hostess as she walked away, ignoring me.

Our server came over and flirted with Kyle and Brendan the entire time she was taking their order.

They both ordered vodka. I ordered a diet Coke.

Even though I had been drinking a lot post-breakup, I didn't know these people that well and didn't want to get drunk at a seedy strip club with a bunch of strangers.

Kyle's drink came out immediately while the rest of us waited fifteen minutes. I rolled my eyes. "Jeez, we get it, he's a good-looking dude. What are we, chopped liver?" I whispered to Katie.

I flagged down our waitress again, "Excuse me, I'm waiting on a Diet Coke. And can we get the wing menu too, please?"

"We don't do wings here anymore. I'll be back with your drink," she said flatly.

Damnit Mother Mary, I had been craving teriyaki for over an hour. My mouth had been salivating at the idea since we left the bar.

This night's a bust, might as well go home and cry myself to sleep, I thought.

The only thing that could redeem the winglessness of this night would be a solid make out session with Kyle.

"So, what are you doing this weekend?" I asked, trying to start a conversation with him.

"You know, playing basketball with some buds. Hitting the gym. Got some Tinder dates," he said.

He wasn't a great conversationalist, but kissing didn't need to involve talking.

"Cool, cool. Where are you going for your dates?"

"Don't know. I'll figure it out later."

I was about to abandon the mission because I obviously wasn't getting anywhere when he casually leaned over, looked at my wrist, and asked, "Is that a watch? It's cool."

It wasn't a watch. It was a Pavlok, a wristband that administers a small electrical shock when touched. It was designed to break bad habits like smoking and nail-biting. I bought it to help me stop touching my hair, a nervous habit that I was trying to break.

Kyle was intrigued by the premise of it.

"What do you mean, it shocks you?" he asked, truly looking at me for the first time all night.

"Well the point is to associate your bad habit with slight pain. It's a way to train yourself to stop associating the habit with pleasure or comfort."

"You shock yourself? Does it hurt?" he asked.

"I mean, it sounds extreme, but it's such a small electrical current. It hurts just enough to make you not want to do the bad habit," I said.

"Can I try it?" His eyes lit up with curiosity and something else I couldn't identify.

"Sure."

I took off the Pavlok and held it against his arm above his wrist. I pressed the button to release the shock. His fist clenched, and his eyes shut in pain.

"Sorry! It can be a lot the first time," I said.

He opened his eyes slowly and, to my surprise, said, "Holy shit. That felt amazing. Do it again, please," closing his eyes in anticipation.

I had let other friends test my Pavlok, but it was the first time anyone had asked for a second go-around. No one had ever claimed it felt good.

I pressed the wristband to his skin and hit the button again. His body shivered in pleasure.

He looked at me with his perfect jaw and his perfect smile and said, "I love it."

A few months earlier I had attended a lecture on fetishes and one of the topics was electroplay, a fetish that involved people receiving a small electric shock during foreplay. I had never heard of it or anything else that involved the word "play" in such a confusing sexual context. It was a little too deep in the kink world for me, but I mentioned it to Kyle.

"Have you ever heard of electroplay? It's a kink. There are safe toys and stuff."

He turned his body to face me and despite being surrounded by half-naked women, I had his undivided attention for a few seconds.

I grabbed my phone and pulled up some forums with toys and explanations of how it worked when Katie stumbled back to our table. She had disappeared for a few minutes and I'd assumed she went to the bathroom.

"C'mon, I bought us both lap dances!" she said, laughing as she approached me, extending her hand to lead me to my dancer.

"What? Why?" I said. I didn't want a lap dance, not to mention, I had just managed to captivate Kyle's attention, I couldn't leave now.

"If we can't have wings, at least we can have lap dances!" she said, grabbing my chair and tilting it to try to make me move.

"No thanks," I said, holding my ground.

"No refunds. C'mon, it will be fun."

"I . . . don't want to do that. . . ." I said as one of the dancers walked over and grabbed my hand. She kissed my cheek and said, "C'mon, baby!" She didn't speak English very well so despite my protests I found myself sitting on one of the leather benches around the perimeter of the club.

There was a tear in the leather next to where I was sitting and I ran my finger across it, trying to figure out what to do.

The dancer straddled me, waving her long, blond hair in my face.

"Hi Sexy, I'm Lexy," she said with a heavy accent, kissing my check, swinging her hair from side to side.

I wasn't drunk enough for this.

"Uh, Olive. Nice to meet you," I stuck out my hand to give her a handshake. I knew it wasn't the right move, but I was unfamiliar with lap dance etiquette.

I turned my head to see what Katie was doing. She was stroking her dancer's back, looking aroused by all of it. It seemed a little *too* comfortable for her.

Lexy started grinding against my leg and I seriously couldn't figure out what the fuck I was supposed to do with my hands. I clasped them awkwardly behind my head like a total bro and didn't touch her at all.

My body was stiff and rigid. I snuck a glance at Kyle who was watching me with bemusement.

I did not sign up for this. All I had wanted was some goddamn wings and to harmlessly flirt with Kyle while I was rebounding.

Lexy unclasped the hook on her purple bikini and pulled it off, waving it in the air. She dragged the fabric across my face and leaned forward.

"You like grills? OPA!" she cried, gyrating against my lap.

I stared at her blankly.

"Grills. Grills? Opa! You like grills?" she said, smiling seductively.

I stared at her for a minute trying to figure out what grilling had to do with any of this when it finally clicked that she meant *girls*.

I thought about it for a second and wanted to launch into a monologue about the Kinsey scale and how there were *some* girls I was attracted to and how my sexuality was a little more fluid than most people's, but I recognized that this wasn't the time or the place, so I just said, "Not really."

She gyrated against my leg while I hardly moved. I couldn't stop giggling, mostly out of nerves but also the ridiculousness of this entire night. I was at a strip club with a bunch of people I barely knew, getting a lap dance and trying to impress a man I didn't want to date with my shock watch.

"So, do you like it here?" I asked, trying to make small talk.

"I'm from the islands!" she replied, smothering my face between her breasts.

The language barrier was obviously not conducive for chatting.

Another giggle escaped my lips as Lexy turned around and rubbed her butt against my stomach, probably so she didn't have to look at me while I was being an uncomfortable weirdo.

"Yeah, baby. Yeah! Opa!" she yelled enthusiastically, swinging her head around so her hair was flying in a circle.

She continued to yell "Opa" and rubbed various parts of her body against mine before releasing me to head back to our table. I didn't know if I was supposed to tip her or not, but I didn't have any cash on me so I just said, "Thank you very much" and walked away.

I saw Katie hand her a ten on my behalf. I'd have to pay her back later.

"You looked so awkward," Kyle said.

"Thanks for pointing it out," I said, taking my seat and grabbing my cola.

The minute I sat down he turned all of his attention back to me and said, "Shock me again. Please. I've never felt anything like that." He held out his wrist.

Happy that this train hadn't been derailed by my abrupt exit, I placed the watch against his skin and watched his face contort with pleasure.

"What does it feel like for you?" I asked, letting my hand linger by his wrist, capitalizing on the fact that I had accidentally discovered a secret toy that aroused the hottest man at the strip club.

"So good," he said.

"Let's try adding something?" I said, reaching up to massage his head with my fingers, stroking gently. "I'm gonna shock you while I rub your head, for different sensations."

"Ready?" I asked.

"Mhhhmm," he said.

He loved it so much that when my island dancer approached him, he declined a lap dance and asked for more shocks instead.

I wanted to believe it was me, but it was definitely the watch. I was making some headway, though.

"I'll be right back. Feel free to use it while I'm gone," I said, getting up to go to the bathroom.

"It's not the same. It's better when you do it to me," he said, flashing his pearly whites. The guy was attractive and he knew it.

I smirked while walking away: my weird sexual knowledge might impress Kyle enough to warrant a kiss at the end of the night.

I walked into a clean one-stall bathroom, thinking about how fascinating it was that Kyle liked being shocked.

I entered the stall, pulled down my pants and found a pool of dark, red blood in the bottom of my underwear.

My period had come.

It hadn't just come, it had come Vin Diesel style, without knocking, busting down the door, and announcing its presence in the most inconvenient way.

I had bled through my underwear and my pants.

I yanked my pants off to see the damage that had been done and saw a grapefruit-sized stain on the back, obvious and dark.

Fuck.

I took off my jacket, tied it around my waist, and hoped it was long enough to cover the stain.

I ran back to my seat, keeping my back to the wall so no one could see my pants. I found an empty table and looked up to see all three members of my party getting lap dances.

I checked my chair for blood and when I didn't see any, I knew that meant one thing.

I had bled all over the lap dance bench.

I thought about pretending that it didn't happen, but it felt unfair to make someone else clean up my blood. Even though periods were totally natural, blood needed to be handled with care.

The lap dance bench was full of gyrating women and hungry clients, but the spot where I had gotten mine was thankfully vacant.

I inched my way closer, trying to examine the bench, hunched over pretending like I had dropped a piece of jewelry. Even though no one was close enough to hear it, I kept saying things like, "oh man, where's my earring?" Finally, when I was about a foot away, I discreetly checked for blood, but I couldn't see any.

A dancer walked by me and when she made eye contact, I said, "Whoops, dropped my earring," and pointed at the floor.

She helped me look and when we couldn't find my non-existent jewelry, I checked the bench again, as best as I could, for blood. It appeared to be blood-free so there was nothing for me to do but high-tail it out of there.

Kyle came back to the table, looking cocky and aroused after his lap dance.

"Hey you, shock me?" he requested.

I was bleeding heavily and in too much of a tizzy to be flirtatious with a boy I had only wanted to make out with.

"I'm so tired," I said, feigning a yawn. "I gotta go." I said. It seemed abrupt because it *was* abrupt. I couldn't sit back in down in my chair because I was afraid of bleeding on it. My only option was to leave as quickly as I could.

"No, don't leave yet," Kyle argued. He wasn't used to women walking away from him. If the circumstances had been different, I might have reveled in that moment of power.

"Sorry, so tired. Really have to go *right now*," I said.

"Shock me one more time," he asked, his eyes almost pleading.

I held out the Pavlok. "Look up electroplay, there are forums and shit," I said before pressing it against his arm, as his eyes rolled back for the umpteenth time.

"Tell Katie and Brendan I said 'bye!'" I yelled, walking out sideways toward the door.

I had to take the subway home because I didn't want to bleed all over the back of a cab. When I got home, I showered, changed into my pajamas and went to bed.

When I woke up in the morning, I felt rough.

After a month of staying out late, drinking too much, and eating crap food, my breakup lifestyle was starting to take a toll on me.

I sat on my couch eating the bacon and eggs I had ordered on Seamless, computer in my lap, scrolling through Facebook.

With a little investigative work, I found Kyle; maybe we could make out a different night.

He was in a relationship.

Of course.

Lindsay walked into the room, took one look at me and said, "Girl, you look like shit. You doin' okay?"

I hadn't seen her in a week. She was in bed by ten when I was getting ready to go out and I woke up after she had already left.

"Yeah, I'm fine. Just busy," I said.

"How's your heart?"

"I've just accepted the fact that I'll probably be alone forever. It's cool."

"You're so dramatic," she said, flicking water at me.

I wiped the water off my face, waited until she was cooking, and said, "Last night I went to a strip club and tried to seduce a man with my shock watch. Then I got my period and bled all over the lap dance bench and had to literally run out the door."

She looked up and caught my eye.

We both burst out laughing, the kind of laughter that you can only have with your best friend without saying anything. I laughed until my stomach hurt and then started again until we were both crying from laughing so hard.

When I was done I said, "Enough. Time to get my shit together."

"Amen, it's time," she said, flipping her eggs.

WHAT IS SEX EVEN?

It was a Saturday morning and I was sitting in a dark warehouse in Brooklyn watching porn with a group of strangers.

It was the second annual Pornfest.

I still wasn't ready to start dating again so I decided to lean in to the "academic side" of my mission to learn about sex. I wasn't sure if Pornfest was technically "academic" but Sheng had invited me to join him and it sounded interesting.

The event was sponsored by YouPorn, one of the largest names in the industry. Because of this, I expected a razzle-dazzle convention with the latest, up-to-date toys and a lot of fanfare.

Yet, the warehouse was dimly lit with only a handful of vendors. There was a stage and a few booths but other than that it was a mild disappointment.

I watched porn. I liked porn. I had my favorite categories (cunnilingus, pegging, and cartoon at the moment) so I was excited to hear from people in the industry. Even though the location was disappointing, the lineup of speakers was pretty good. I had just watched a panel with three camgirls and took notes the whole time.

Next up was Cindy Gallop, the founder of MakeLoveNotPorn, a social site with real people having real sex. "Let me be clear. We are pro-sex, pro-porn, pro-education," Cindy said, brushing her electric blond hair out of her face. She was the reason most of the audience was there. She was a brilliant speaker and a charismatic woman in her fifties, not to mention. sexy as hell.

Cindy looked at the audience, pointing her microphone upward, "The issue is that we, as a society, don't talk about sex," she said.

Amen, sister.

If I wasn't proof of that then I didn't know what or who was.

"What we do at MakeLoveNotPorn is offer the opportunity to watch *real* couples having *real* sex. I could explain it, or I could show you," Cindy said with a smile.

Suddenly the screen lit up with a couple, naked and joking about what sex toys they liked.

I had only ever watched porn in private, with headphones, so my roommates wouldn't have any idea what I was up to. The idea of watching it together with a room full of people was both exciting and scary.

I was sitting next to Sheng; his unruly brown hair was longer than normal. I was worried that I'd get turned on and he'd somehow sense it. The idea of being aroused in a room full of people still felt uncomfortable to me.

The woman on screen put on a strap-on. She fumbled and dropped it at one point, which I guess is what Cindy meant by real sex.

I *was* aroused, but somehow it was different than what I expected. It wasn't making me so horny that I wanted to hump the closest thing I could find. Instead it was making me crave human connection. I wanted to reach over and touch Sheng's hand but I knew that was inappropriate. Instead I tried to sit as still as a I possibly could, lest my movement give away any signs of arousal.

After the screening, we took a break and I meandered over to a vibrator table. I was holding a large, purple dildo when I bumped into another writer I knew.

"Good to see you, darling! What are you doing here?" she asked.

"Aw, you know, research and stuff," I replied, leaning in to give her a hug.

She introduced me to another writer, Jane, that she had worked with before.

"Nice to meet you, what do you write about?" Jane asked. I used my classic line, explaining that I was exploring sex after a five-year dry spell, which, thank God, I had broken earlier that year.

"You haven't been with anyone in five years?" she asked.

"Well, I mean, I've been with people but no actual sex."

"What do you mean by actual sex?"

I explained that there had been oral, mutual masturbation, and tons of orgasms during the dry spell, but no penis in my vagina.

"Then you've had sex," she said.

I started to protest when she said, "So when my girlfriend and I make love to each other, we aren't having sex?"

I had never thought of it like that. She had a point. Of course they were having sex.

"Do you masturbate?" she prompted.

"Yes."

"That's sex. You've had sex."

My seventh-grade sex ed class had always defined sex as a penis entering a vagina, but it was clear that that definition was limiting and inaccurate for so many couples.

Also, when I was in seventh grade, Pluto was still a planet. Times had changed.

I excused myself, deeply embarrassed by my exclusionary language.

I returned to my seat and typed "What is sex?" into the Google search engine on my phone.

I was thirty years old and had just spent the last year examining my own sexuality, and yet my search history clearly revealed how much further I had to go.

"Sex means different things to different people," the first website said.

Well, that wasn't helpful.

Was I the only one with this question? Was everyone else clear on how to define sex? What counted and what didn't? By the time the next panel came on, I was deep down the rabbit hole, reading about the Mormon practice of "Floating" which involved inserting the penis but not moving it. According to Floating practitioners, moving counted as sex. There were also the high schoolers having anal sex who claimed it didn't count and the "just-the-tippers" who also asserted it wasn't "officially" sex.

While I was Googling, I also discovered that I had been using the term vagina wrong this whole time. A vagina was actually the term for the inside, and what you could see on the outside was the vulva. I was still learning things I should have known by then.

What was sex, even?

For five years I'd claimed I was celibate, but was I?

I wasn't sure anymore because I couldn't even figure out what sex was and wasn't able to properly name the parts of my own anatomy.

I couldn't come up with any sort of definitive answer and wasn't sure I was ever going to. Instead, I returned to my seat to collectively watch porn and try too hard not to seem aroused.

CLARK KENT

Summer had turned into fall and fall into cuffing season when I started chatting with Amit on Facebook Messenger. Amit was blind date number ten, a date I never went on because I started seeing Simon. We had been chatting online, like it was 1994, for a few weeks now.

Amit was six feet tall with dark skin, deep brown eyes, and an impeccable fashion sense. He was one of the only men I knew who wore hats remarkably well, at least according to his Facebook profile.

"So, you're single again?" he asked one day.

"Yep," I replied.

"Let's go on that date," he said.

I was looking forward to going out with him because I enjoyed our online rapport and was excited to see if it translated into real life.

For our first date, we met up at a fancy sushi restaurant where he showed up looking hot as hell in a dark blue suit.

Unfortunately, as soon as we sat down, we struggled to find things to talk about and had long, unbearable pauses. After we ordered, he showed me a hundred pictures of his cat and when he dropped his fork, he said "Cheese sticks!" instead of "shit." On paper it sounds endearing, but I wasn't into it at all.

We had nothing in common, and I was disappointed that our online rapport did *not* translate into real life.

When he offered to walk me to the train, I figured it was our first and last date. I assumed we were on the same page, so I was surprised when he kissed me at the end of it. I was even more surprised by how good it was. For all his awkwardness, Amit knew how to kiss.

First dates aren't always great, so I wanted to give him a second chance. On our second date we went for tacos and got a little too drunk on margaritas. The alcohol made him chattier and by the end of the night, I was having a good time. We went back to his place, made out like teenagers, got partially naked, and fooled around.

One thing became pretty clear: Amit was savvy in the sack.

He was a total Clark Kent in real life and a Superman when he was about to get naked.

Amit made no effort to schedule a third date, a fact that both annoyed me and didn't bother me at all. When he finally scheduled it, it was almost a month later and Christmas season in NYC. We went to see the tree at Rockefeller Center. Once again, we were struggling to find things to talk about. We ordered hot cocoa and held hands through our mittens but by his seventy-fifth pun, I was ready to leave.

I planned on going home, alone, until he kissed me with one of his soul-melting, voodoo-magic, where-did-that-come-from kisses. I decided to go to his place instead.

We hopped on the subway and rode the train together silently. I rubbed his leg because touch was the only common language that we shared.

In that moment, I realized two things:

1. I did not want to date him, but . . .
2. I wanted to keep fooling around with him.

We couldn't date because we had nothing to talk about, he was obsessed with his cat, and his dad humor was seriously grating on my nerves.

My friends thought Amit sounded great. *They* didn't get a friend request from Prince Oscar of Kittenville, his cat's private Instagram account.

And yet, somehow, our bodies responded to each other.

Usually if I wasn't interested emotionally, I wasn't interested physically.

Not with Amit. Must have had something to do with pheromones and biology.

And sexts.

Amit was a top-notch sexter. I have no idea how it started, but we were sexting after our first date. It felt too-soon and also thrilling. His sexts were graphic yet respectful. Dirty without crossing any lines. He'd send pictures of his abs (no face, of course) with a list of all the things he wanted to do to me. I'd ask if he was aroused and if he said "yes" I'd say "Show me" and he'd send bathroom photos of his erection. It was all very exciting. Even though our in-person dates weren't magical, when we kissed, I think we both mentally traveled to the digital version of the other person.

It was weird, in real life, he was this handsome nerdy dude who had zero game. Over text, or if he was about to fool around, he was this nasty sex machine.

When we arrived at his house after our Rockefeller Center date, he made me watch a dance he had choreographed with Prince Oscar and then turned on *A Charlie Brown Christmas.*

Thirty minutes into Linus and Lucy and I was bored out of my fucking mind. I couldn't figure out why he wasn't making a move.

"Look, they have another Christmas special, I haven't seen this one!" he said with almost childlike excitement when the first one ended.

I didn't want to burst his bubble, but there was no way in hell I was about to sit through another Charlie Brown special. That's the kind of shit you do by yourself, when you've already watched *Game of Thrones* and literally everything else. We were doing too much Netflixing and too little chilling.

I had to take action.

I pulled the remote out of his hand and straddled him.

"I'd rather do this," I said, leaning in to kiss him.

"Better idea," he agreed, wrapping my legs around him.

Superman was back.

He picked me up and carried me to the bed with a level of assertion that he reserved for sexy times.

He pulled my shirt over my head in one swift motion before pulling his own off.

"Kiss me now," I demanded, wrapping my arms around his neck.

He kissed me hard, moving his tongue in and out of my mouth with expertise before kissing my face and my cheek.

"I'm gonna make you cum multiple times," he said confidently as he unfastened my bra.

This was the same guy who choregraphed dances with his cats?

"Oh yeah? How?" Both of our bodies were starting to get hot.

"Like this," he said, rolling me over and kissing me firmly down my body.

I wasn't planning on having sex with Amit, but he was true to his word. After three orgasms, I was gasping for breath and clinging to his body.

"Get a condom," I said, digging my nails into his back.

We had sex that was both gentle and, at times, aggressive, talking dirty the whole time, our texting conversations becoming real life.

Amit changed positions with ease and the sex was seamless in a way I hadn't ever experienced.

My body was doing all the work and, thank God, my brain decided it needed a break.

When we finished, we cuddled for an hour and then started round two.

"Holy shit," I said, breathless and sweaty when everything was done.

He got up, went to the bathroom, picked up Prince Oscar, and started dancing with him.

Just like that, Clark Kent made his return.

"Want to watch the second Charlie Brown?" he asked, plopping down on the couch.

I definitely did not want to do that.

"Oh, I mean I should probably get going," I said, pulling on my jeans.

I kissed him passionately, pet Prince Oscar a few times, and then walked down the hall toward the elevator.

As the elevator raced toward the ground floor, I caught a glimpse of my reflection in the doors.

My hair was messy. My face was glowing. I was carrying my shoes and wearing the backup flats I had stashed in my purse. I started to untangle my hair, smoothing down strays with a quick spit-lick.

Another woman entered the elevator and smirked at me.

Suddenly it dawned on me: I was doing a Walk of Shame.

Holy shit, me, the leading damsel of chastity, was doing my first-ever Walk of Shame! I went through the events of the evening in my mind:

I had slept with a man on the third date.

We had tried four different positions in one night.

They had all felt amazing.

I did not stay the night.

Me. Someone who always stayed the night.

Who was I?

The best part was that I didn't feel the constant nagging guilt that I thought I would feel. I felt totally fine about all of it. I'd had sex. *Because I wanted to.*

For me, that was huge. Usually there was an entire melodrama of emotions and inner monologues with fear and insecurity as the leading directors.

I stopped trying to smooth out my hair. To hell with it. I'd just come from a man's apartment and I wasn't ashamed.

In fact, I was a little bit proud of myself.

I had come a long way.

THE FRIENDS WITH
BENEFITS EXPERIMENT

I got the idea for the Friends with Benefits Experiment from an article I had read on the Internet.

It was called, "How Deepening Friends with Benefits Led Me to Love." It told the story of a man, Andrew, who entered into a thoughtful and intentional "friends with benefits" situation with a woman, Dana. They set guidelines and rules (like no going on dates, texting, etc.) and promised to communicate honestly. Their experiment allowed them to openly and vulnerably explore sexuality. Andrew and Dana both married other people but credited their FWB experiment for teaching them how to embrace intimacy and love.

Hmm, that sounded nice. If only I had someone to . . .

Amit.

He was the perfect person to experiment with. I was still feeling self-conscious about my sexual prowess and Amit made things easy. Our chemistry was strong enough that I wasn't overanalyzing or judging myself. It was low-stakes sex with someone I trusted without the emotional roller coaster I'd had with Simon.

With Simon, I was too uncertain about our relationship to ever be fully relaxed with him in the bedroom.

I sent the article to Amit, and then outright asked him if he wanted to try being my FWB. I hadn't heard from him in two weeks, so I was pretty sure he didn't want to date me either.

"I'm still newish to all this, so it might be fun," I said.

"I'm down like a rodeo clown!" he responded.

I didn't know what that meant but it was a very Amit thing to say.

We met up for coffee the next day and talked about the guidelines. I had a Friend with Benefits in college, but I had never talked about boundaries and explorations beforehand. It was a smart thing to do, since it's pretty hard to have that conversation once everyone was naked.

I looked at him over my latte and noticed how handsome he looked. I didn't know how to start so I smiled and said, "What are you hoping to get from this?"

"Well, I haven't had the opportunity to explore like this and you've been researching sex for a while, so I'd love to learn new ways to pleasure you and receive pleasure," he answered. "What about you?"

"Same. Sort of. I mean, basically I want to feel like a confident and competent lover."

"You are already all of those things."

"Thank you," I said, taking a sip from my mug so he wouldn't see me blush. "I just want to feel that way, though." I continued, "What do you need out of this, like guidelines, I mean?"

"Safety. I mean we need to always be safe and if you decide to take on other partners, let me know, and vice versa," he responded.

We established that first and foremost, we'd be honest with each other at all times.

We'd be considerate, thoughtful, and safe partners always.

"I want to kiss and cuddle afterward and not make it weird," I said. I knew I needed affection or else I would start to feel crappy and cheap about the whole thing.

We agreed that our aftercare (how you treated your partner after sex) might involve cuddling and leaving or occasionally staying over. We wouldn't make it awkward either way.

We also agreed that we weren't accountable to each other outside of the bedroom. He didn't owe me a "How is your day?" text and we were both free agents, able to date as we pleased.

Now it was time for the fun part. We were both going to make a list of things we wanted to try.

I pulled two pieces of paper out of my backpack that I had printed from the Internet. They were "Yes, No, Maybe" lists. On each side, there were categories of things to try sexually. We'd each fill it out, placing a Yes, No, or Maybe next to each suggestion, indicating whether or not we wanted to try it. Then we would exchange lists.

I grabbed a book to write on and hid my list under the table and started filling it out.

Blindfolds. Yes.

Body Paint. Yes.

Double Penetration. No.

Food Play. Yes.

Saran Wrap. Maybe? I guess it would depend on the context.

I filled out my list and waited until Amit was done with his and then we exchanged them.

His list included things like: Prostate massage, anal play, role-playing, and threesomes. Mine included pegging, role-playing, BDSM, and watching porn together.

Because I didn't want to date Amit, there was no fear of rejection. Since there was no fear of rejection, we were able to reveal our desires honestly.

I wanted to give us both time to think about our arrangement and see if anything else came up before we put our plan into action, so we agreed to meet the following Saturday.

On Thursday, Amit sent me a Snapchat of his erection at work with the text, "Thinking of you."

We met on the street three hours later, kissing each other with intensity and need. We made small talk but we weren't trying too hard to be funny or impressive.

When we got to his house, he asked, "What do you want and what do you need?"

"I want you and I need a shoulder massage, badly," I said, partially joking.

"Let me massage you. Undress and lay down," he instructed.

I lay down in his bed completely naked, all my "problem-areas" out in the open, without any desire to hide them under a sheet.

He gently massaged my shoulders, using his thumbs around the knots in my neck. He spent a long time there, alternating between light and heavy touches. He moved his hands down my back, following my instructions of "right there" and "harder." He was taking his time.

He moved to my butt and kissed each cheek before massaging muscles I didn't even know I had.

With my other lovers, sex had felt linear.

It was always oral sex followed by vaginal sex. Cuddle. The end.

Foreplay felt like something you did on the way to penetrative sex. Everything that happened along the way was cursory. With Amit, there was no final destination. Our only "goal" was to figure out what made the other person squirm, to enjoy the other person's body. There was no expectation of sex from either side. Foreplay for the sake of foreplay was such a fun and delicious game.

Since there wasn't a final destination, Amit took his time, rubbing my back for a full half an hour. He was sensual and slow, massaging my thighs and my arms. He never tried to hurry things along or seemed like he was doing it out of obligation.

When he was done, I sighed happily.

I knew I should return the favor, and probably would have if we were dating, but I didn't want to give him a backrub. That was the best thing about a Friend with Benefits, nothing needed to be tit-for-tat.

Instead I leaned over his chest and licked his nipple with my tongue.

He moaned slightly and rubbed my arm while I took his nipple in my mouth, flicking it softly.

"Stay there, please," he said. One of our agreements was that we would ask for what we wanted.

I kept my mouth around his nipple for a long time, sucking it. Nibbling on it gently. In any other scenario, it might have seemed like forever but since it wasn't a means to an end, we were both enjoying it.

I moved on to his other nipple and pinched it lightly and then roughly.

"Which do you prefer?" I asked.

"Pinch it hard," he said.

I pinched his nipple harder, alternating between that and strokes from my tongue.

Effortlessly, in one motion, he flipped me over and mirrored what I had just done to him on my own nipples.

Without haste, he kissed his way down to my pussy. As his warm tongue landed on my clitoris, I moaned with pleasure.

He alternated between rubbing it with two fingers and licking it until I was on the brink of an orgasm. Then with expertise, he increased the pacing until I came.

He wasn't done. He moved back to my nipples, rubbing his finger across each one, slowly, until I arched my back up to meet him.

He kissed me passionately before returning back to my clit for round two.

My body responded immediately.

"Your neighbors are going to hate you," I joked between moans.

"Mmhhhmm," he replied, his mouth too busy for words.

In a few minutes, I had my second orgasm and melted into his bed.

We lay there cuddling and spooning for a long time, running our hands all over each other, making jokes and being silly about what turned us on.

Pretending to be a cat, I swatted his arm and "meowed," playfully teasing him. "Seriously though, do you know how many cat videos you made me watch? What is up with that?"

"My cat is awesome. The world needs to know."

If we were trying to date, I would have sucked it up and watched a zillion more cat videos and never said anything. The ability to be honest was exactly what made the whole arrangement beneficial. We could say what we were thinking.

"But three videos on one date? I mean . . ."

He leaned into his best line of defense, cutting me off by stroking me from behind.

"It's too . . ." I was incapable of finishing the sentence because I was moaning louder than before, the pleasure rippling down my body.

"The world must know about my cat," he said, grinning devilishly at his own ability to make me stop talking.

In seconds, I came for the third time that night.

I felt feral, like a wild animal. Uncontrolled. I was the embodiment of unbridled sexuality.

I bit him, hard, on his shoulder.

"You're my bad, bad Superman," I said, showering his body with kisses and nips.

I rolled over and took his erection in my mouth, sloppily and with enthusiasm.

When he was moaning the same way I had, I said, "Get a condom."

I hadn't stayed over with the intention of having sex that night, but my God did I want to.

He hopped out of bed and was back before I even noticed he was gone. I reached for him hungrily.

He grabbed my ankles with the same need and held them up in the air, pushing my legs back toward my face before immediately entering me.

He thrust quickly and rapidly. It was the perfect amount of aggression after hours of sensual slowness.

He ejaculated quickly and collapsed. We lay there for a while, breathing erratically before he said, "You're hot," meaning temperature-wise; I was burning up.

He propped himself up on his side and started blowing across my body, like someone would do with soup, trying to cool me down. It was such a thoughtful gesture. He could have rolled away, too engrossed in his own orgasm, but instead he was still trying to make sure I was comfortable and taken care of. It was too bad we weren't compatible for dating.

We cuddled for another hour, touching and holding each other before I got up to leave. He invited me to stay for dinner, but I was too afraid he had the Charlie Brown New Year's special cued up and ready to go.

Besides, we were better in bed than out of it.

I didn't text him later and he didn't text me. I didn't dream or fantasize about him, but it also wasn't lost on me that our ability to be vulnerable and honest with each other was allowing us to have incredible sex.

The next time I saw him, I brought my rope from the BDSM class. I tied him up and made him call me Mistress. I never once said please as I tried to recreate the sexiness I felt with the Irishman. It wasn't hard, since I was good at bossing people around.

We both enjoyed ourselves and agreed that maybe next time we'd explore some toy stuff. I couldn't believe it, but this Friend with Benefits thing was working out.

I was starting to feel like maybe I knew what I was doing.

A CUDDLING CATASTROPHE

February arrived with a vengeance and with it, the kind of chill that freezes your bones. On a particularly cold NYC night I was sitting on my couch at 2 a.m. wrapped in a blanket, thinking about what I wanted in that exact moment.

I wanted winter to be over. I wanted to magically snap my fingers and have a bowl of soup without having to make soup. I wanted warmer socks and three more episodes of *The Unbreakable Kimmy Schmidt*.

Mostly, I wanted a warm body next to mine to cuddle away the cold. I pulled up Amit's number.

"Come cuddle," I started texting, but I stopped before I could send it. It was late and my relationship with Amit was purely physical, and it worked that way. Asking him to come over to cuddle at 2 a.m. would have infringed on the terms of our FWB situation. Also, I knew it would have turned into something more than cuddling. I realized that although Amit was fulfilling a necessary role, all of my needs weren't being met. The problem: I wanted affection without sex. To be held by someone without having to do anything else.

A hundred percent just cuddling.

I tapped my finger on the keyboard, brainstorming a solution.

Because it was late, and I was delirious, I pulled up Google and typed "Platonic cuddling" in the search bar, just to see if anything would pop up. I had no expectations, but New York's full of surprises.

The first website that came up was called the Cuddling Cave. It was a free site, similar to OKCupid, for people looking for "cuddles only."

I clicked on it. The home page raved about the effects of cuddling on the brain and the dopamine spikes caused by human touch.

They didn't have to convince me. I knew how weird and desperate a person became when they were hungry for touch.

Before Simon, I was starving.

I scrolled through some of the profiles and decided to join, because, why not? I had nothing to lose. I uploaded a picture and filled in my profile with one sentence.

"Smart, funny, and kind: looking for JUST cuddling." It was my laziest, bare-minimum effort. I went to bed and buried myself under three blankets, fantasizing about a pajama-clad man next to me.

The next morning, I woke up to twenty-five messages in my cuddle inbox. Apparently, my laziest, bare-minimum effort was enough when the ratio of men to women was thirty to one.

My chat box lit up as a man messaged me in real time, "Price? In-call only?"

Oh, I thought.

This site was actually for people trying to buy sex. I should have known that "platonic cuddling" wasn't a real thing.

I messaged him back, "I thought this site was for *just* cuddling? What are you paying for? What's an in-call?"

"Yeah, you're paying for cuddling. Lots of professional cuddlers on here, they charge an hourly rate. In-call means we cuddle at your place, out-call means we cuddle at my place," he replied.

"Cool, thanks! Not for hire though," I wrote back.

I scanned through some women's profiles and found a lot of "certified" professional cuddlers offering "touch therapy" to a whole slew of happy clients. They charged sixty to eighty dollars an hour. Their profiles emphasized things like Egyptian sheets and rooms with air purifiers.

I wasn't interested in hiring someone or being hired, so I scanned back to my messages, to find someone who didn't want to pay me. My eyes landed on a message from a hot guy with a neatly-trimmed beard, playing the trumpet.

His name was Steve. He was twenty-four and according to his message, had cuddled with three people on the site and had an "absolute blast."

We arranged to meet up later that week.

In person, he looked like his picture: average height with a dark reddish beard and a cleft chin. We hugged and I noticed, with delight, that he smelled like oranges. We decided to go on a walk and thank goodness, it had gotten slightly warmer, though I was still wearing my winter coat and snow boots.

We chatted about ourselves for a little bit (he was a former band-nerd, I was a former theater nerd. We both liked ramen and Broadway shows) before moving on to cuddling.

As the practiced cuddler, Steve took the lead, answering my questions.

And I had a lot of questions.

Like how the hell did it work?

What did people wear? When did they leave? Was it truly cuddling or were people using it as a way to find sex?

He answered my questions with authority. People wore pajamas or whatever they wanted. They left when they were done. It was *mostly* just cuddling.

He had a few other cuddling buddies and raved about how much cuddling had improved his life and self-image. Like me, he was overweight as a teen and still getting used to his new body. Cuddling had taught him to be more comfortable in his own skin.

I was digging his vibe, flirting and touching his arm.

When I told him I was writing a book, he said, "Are you going to put cuddling in it?"

"I don't know, maybe," I said. "I messaged you because I wanted someone to cuddle with, not for a story."

He asked me what else I'd done. I began telling him about tickling but I stopped halfway. I have a tendency to prematurely overshare.

"I shouldn't tell you this," I said.

"Of course you should. Let's be clear; we're not on a date. I'm not looking for a relationship. This is purely platonic cuddling, so you don't have to worry about impressing me and vice versa." Steve was a programmer and it became clear he operated from a place of logic. Everything he said was direct and straightforward.

I appreciated the clarity in that moment and dropped the flirtatious fakeness I adopt when I'm trying too hard. I didn't have to be cute, or pretty, or interesting. I told him about tickling, my fears around sex, and why I was doing all of this in the first place.

He asked if anything about cuddling scared me. Since we weren't trying to date, I answered bluntly, telling him that I was afraid he'd rape or kill me and that no one would believe me because I met him on a cuddling site.

He looked taken aback before answering dismissively, "That makes no sense. You know who my employer is." I had to laugh that *that* was somehow supposed to reassure me.

We walked around for another thirty minutes before sitting down on some steps, brushing off the snow.

"So, what do you think? Wanna cuddle?" he asked, blowing into his gloves to warm his hands.

I tightened my scarf around my neck and weighed the pros and cons.

Pros: Cuddling with a good-smelling, attractive man.

Cons: He might kill me.

"Let's do this," I said.

And to think, I used to be so cautious. Now I'd become someone who invited strangers from the Internet over to cuddle. My dad would kill me.

Even though he lived closer, I insisted we go to my house because my roommates were home, which meant I could potentially call for help in case he *did* turn out to be a serial killer.

Lindsay and Mary were sitting on the couch when we walked in watching the season finale of *Big Brother*.

I didn't make any excuses. "This is Steve, we're going to platonically cuddle," I said.

They didn't bat an eye. They were used to my shenanigans by that point.

Steve chatted with them for ten minutes, which was nice and odd at the same time. Like he said, we weren't on a date. There was no need to be overly friendly with my roommates.

"Let's go," I said, grabbing his hand and leading him down the hallway to my room. When we got there, I wasn't sure what to do.

Lights on? Lights off?

Over the covers? Under?

Steve took the lead and laid down on top of my sheets, fully clothed. I decided on lights off and laid down next to him, stiff as a board, my arm draped over his chest.

Through my window, I could hear the sounds of car sirens below. One of my neighbors was blasting some old-school Nelly. Beyond that, the room was silent.

We lay there quietly for what seemed like forever before I could fully relax. I took in a deep breath, trying to calm myself and let my body sink in next to his. He reached over, grabbed a piece of my hair and started twirling it around his finger.

"You smell amazing," he said too loudly. The volume was jarring in contrast to the silence in the room.

"Thank you," I whispered back.

It was supposed to be platonic, but our rising body temperature made it clear that it wasn't. We were attracted to each other and while cuddling was nice, we were both trying to get as close as possible.

"I'm getting a little hot, do you mind if I take my shirt off?" he asked.

That was dangerous. I didn't want it to escalate but I also thought about how nice it would be to touch his skin directly.

My dopamine-soaked brain won, and I said, "Sure."

I ran my hand over his body, softly playing with his chest hair.

My cheek was resting against his collarbone, my breath coming out hot over his chest and while I knew I shouldn't do it, should have tried harder to stop myself, I couldn't resist flicking my tongue across his nipple.

He let out a deep, guttural groan.

For someone who had been celibate for five years, I was demonstrating remarkably low self-control.

I wanted to take off my shirt too, to feel his skin against mine.

I was crossing a line. I knew it, but the sweater in-between us felt like a concrete partition.

"Would you mind if I take my shirt off, too?"

"Be my guest," he said.

I pulled my sweater off over my head and laid next to him in my bra.

"My God, you're magnificent," he said, his eyes full of desire as he grazed my breasts with his eyes.

Damnit, I was a sucker for compliments. I still wasn't used to people telling me I was beautiful, so compliments melted my willpower more than any other drug.

He caressed my arm while I nuzzled my head in his neck. We were escalating the intensity, touching and responding to each other without making it overtly sexual.

He moved quickly and was on top of me, grinding his hips into mine, raising and lowering his pelvis against me, aggressively dry humping me.

I hadn't been dry humped in years.

I was about to tell him to knock it off when he yelled loudly and stopped.

"I just came," he said.

I looked down and saw a wet spot on his sweatpants. I hadn't seen anyone cum in their pants in over a decade. I wasn't sure if I should laugh or get pissed off.

It had happened in less than thirty seconds, which left me bewildered by the whole situation. We hadn't even kissed.

"I'm gonna go clean up," he said, heading to the bathroom.

I sat up, trying to sort through the emotions I was feeling. I was confused about what had happened. Aroused by the closeness of his body. Angry that he had used my body to cum without my consent, even if it was just dry humping. Then again, it was in his pants, so I guess it was harmless. And I probably shouldn't have taken off my shirt or licked his nipple. Then again, he shouldn't have humped me. Was he in the wrong? Had I encouraged it? Was I in the wrong?

The whole situation was bizarre, and I couldn't make heads or tails of it.

I was still waffling over these emotions when he left. We didn't kiss or hug but waved to each other on the way out. I told Lindsay about it the next morning and she was as baffled as I was. She said he gave her a weird vibe and she wasn't surprised.

He texted me the next day to set up another cuddling session. That's what we were calling them, apparently: "sessions."

If by session he meant "cuddle and then I'm going to cum in my pants while dry humping you," then I didn't want to. I probably should have told him to buzz off, but I didn't because despite being annoyed, I kept remembering the look on his face when he said, "You're magnificent."

I had to put my foot down and set a clear boundary.

"We crossed lines we shouldn't have crossed. I'm not looking for a Friend with Benefits," I wrote. I already had Amit and I was satisfied with that situation. Two Friends with Benefits was way too much.

If Steve couldn't be my cuddle buddy, then it was on to another message in my inbox.

"We'll just cuddle this time. Last time was an anomaly. We'll set a timer and everything," he promised.

He came up to Harlem three days later and I told him the new rules, which someone had suggested on the Cuddling Cave website. We'd set an alarm for forty-five minutes and cuddle fully clothed over the covers. No kissing. No nipple-touching. Definitely no orgasming.

Platonic.

I laid down next to him, the sound of my heart thudding in my ears. I focused on my breathing, in and then out. In and then out. Eventually, I entered a meditative state where I was relaxed and comfortable. I was experiencing the "feel-good" chemicals the website had gone on and on about.

By the time the alarm went off, I was almost asleep.

We took our time sitting up, peaceful smiles on our faces. This was exactly what I had been looking for. We had been successfully platonic, and I felt amazing, like I'd gone to the spa, done yoga, and slept for twelve hours.

We platonically cuddled again two more times before he started texting me daily.

I didn't have time to cuddle more than once a week, a fact that he was disappointed about.

"Why don't you call your other cuddle buddies?" I offered, trying to be helpful.

"I want to cuddle with *you*. I can't stop thinking about it," he said.

We scheduled another appointment for the following week. Amit had been MIA for two weeks now, so I was looking forward to seeing Steve.

I set the alarm and snuggled into his chest, breathing in the scent of his cologne, listening to his heart beat.

Instead of relaxing into a meditative state, I could feel our body heat rising.

I had set strict rules for good reasons. It had worked for three sessions.

The alarm buzzed, I silenced it, and returned my head back to Steve's chest. Neither one of us moved.

He ran a finger along my collarbone.

"You have the most perfect body I've ever seen," he said.

He always managed to melt my resistance with his damn compliments. How was a lady supposed to restrain herself when a gent was bathing her in such lovely accolades?

I looked at him for a moment and decided to break my own carefully crafted rules. I was tired of being someone who made arbitrary rules and then felt guilty for breaking them, when no one but me even cared at all.

"I don't want a Friend with Benefits," I said.

"I know."

"But I also want to kiss you right now."

He looked surprised.

"I want to kiss you, but I don't want to set a precedent. I love cuddling with you. Sometimes I'm going to just want that. So, if I kiss you right now, can we agree that sometimes we kiss and sometimes we're platonic, but we'll always discuss it clearly?" I asked.

He agreed.

Clothing came off as he kissed downward toward my thigh. I wasn't ready for oral sex. We hadn't discussed our sexual history and it felt too intimate.

I still wanted to fool around, though, so I caressed his body before positioning his dick firmly between my breasts, using my arm to squeeze them together for extra pressure. I moved my breasts up and down until I was certain he was going to wake all of my neighbors with his moans. He came, strongly and fiercely.

Into his own eye.

I marveled for a minute at his utterly inconvenient aim and the white liquid coating his left eyelid.

He leapt out of bed, jumping around, screaming, "It's in my eye. Fuck! Fuck! I gotta clean it before I get pink eye."

I scrunched my eyelids together, "What does that have to do with pink eye?" I asked.

In a panic, he told me about a time at summer camp when a fellow camper got it and the counselor told them that pink eye was caused by cum. He had been afraid ever since, frantically washing his hands every time he jerked off.

I couldn't help myself, laughing lightly at first as he rushed off to the bathroom. By the time Steve returned from the bathroom, I was on the ground, incapable of breathing because I was laughing so hard.

"Wait, you think that pink eye . . . is only . . . caused by . . ." I couldn't finish my sentence.

I doubled over in another round of laughter at this revelation. I imagined him hearing that a fifty-year-old coworker was out because of conjunctivitis and thinking, "She got jizz in her eye!"

I waited until I could talk and gently explained that pink eye wasn't always a direct correlation to cum in the eye.

"Are you sure?"

"Yes," I said.

Still giggling, I sat down on the bed beckoning him to come join me.

He sat down next to me. "I've never orgasmed like that in my whole life," he said stroking my hair. "My body responds to you in ways I don't understand."

I thought about everything I knew about Steve. He was young and had told me he didn't talk to women until late adolescence. He alluded to the fact that he was a sexual veteran, but all evidence pointed elsewhere. As much I wanted to believe I was a sex deity who turned men's bodies to mush, it seemed more plausible that Steve was more inexperienced than I was. For the first time in my life, I was the one with more sexual competence.

I invited him to stay the night but he said he couldn't sleep with someone else in a bed and he needed a good night's sleep, so he left and headed home.

I ran into Mary in the hall, on her way to use the bathroom.

"Heard Steve. Are you guys, like, dating now?" she asked, yawning, her eyes only half open.

"I mean no. We're . . . doing a thing? We're cuddle buddies?"

I tried to think of the right title but I couldn't because what we were doing was abnormal, we weren't exactly cuddle buddies anymore but we also weren't Friends with Benefits.

I turned to the Internet for help and typed, "What do you call someone you sometimes platonically cuddle with and sometimes fool around with but don't have sex with?" My fellow Interneters were as confused as I was, commenting "That's not a thing." and "It's called a clusterfuck, and I agree, not a thing."

A few weeks later, Steve left for Florida. To my surprise, I missed him. Amit was still mysteriously MIA and I was craving affection.

In truth, I was craving Steve.

I looked up "cuddling" to see if anything came up about it being addictive.

Turns out it was.

According to Google, cuddling was biologically addictive because it caused the brain to release oxytocin, which makes someone feel more loving toward their partner. Couples who cuddled could feel withdrawal symptoms when their partner was gone thanks to the reduction of oxytocin.

I texted him the sentiment, "I'm going through withdrawal."

"You have no idea what that does to my body," he wrote back.

I had a little bit of an idea.

"I think I like you," he said.

"I think I might like you too," I replied.

"Let's go on a real date when I get back?" he asked.

"I'd like that," I said.

We met up at an Italian restaurant for our first actual date and he was standing inside waiting for me to arrive.

"Hi!" I said leaning in to kiss him.

He turned his head. "Oh, I don't do PDA. Kissing should be reserved for the bedroom, unless you're already boyfriend and girlfriend," he said with as much self-assuredness as he said everything.

I stared at him, realizing that even though I'd seen the man cum in his own eye, there was still a hell of a lot I didn't know about him.

The date was going well enough. I could ignore the fact that Steve chewed with his mouth open and acted like he was the expert in literally everything, but things took a turn when I told him about one of my other experiences on Cuddling Cave.

I had gotten a message from a man who ultimately confessed that he had lied about his age and used a fake profile picture. It turned out he was in his fifties and married. Instead of apologizing for deceiving me, he acted like I should cuddle with him anyway.

"He was probably very lonely," Steve interjected aggressively, as if I was confronting him personally.

I couldn't figure out why he was defending this nameless, faceless man on the Internet over taking my side.

"Of course," I replied. "I can empathize with that, but loneliness doesn't give you the right to be deceitful."

"Well we can't all be young, thirty, and beautiful," he said resentfully.

I stared at him for a moment, alarmed that he was directing his anger at me. What annoyed me the most was the implication that this man's loneliness was somehow my responsibility and therefore entitled him with access to my body. I could empathize with the problem, but I didn't have to be the solution.

"You think I don't understand what it feels like to think no one is ever going to touch you?" I asked pointedly.

"Well, good-looking women usually don't have that problem," he muttered.

I pulled out a picture of me from when I was younger and shoved it in his face.

"I know what it's like to feel undesirable. Still doesn't give you the right to lie."

We ate in silence for a few minutes and when the waitress walked by I asked for our check.

We both went home alone.

The next morning he texted, "I'm sorry about yesterday. That guy shouldn't have lied to you and I shouldn't have defended him."

I didn't respond and an hour later he wrote, "Look, I can't explain it, but I'm infatuated with you and I hate it because I hate feeling out of control. Why do I respond to you the way I do? It doesn't make sense and I like it when things make sense. I like order and you're chaos and I want you more than I have ever wanted anyone."

He was Christian Greying me.

Talking about how much he needed and wanted me, making me feel powerful, and sexy, like there was something uniquely special about only me that made him go crazy with desire.

As ashamed as I am to admit it, I fell for it.

We had a few good "sessions" or dates or whatever we were calling them after that. Usually we met up at his place, cuddled, did some light fooling around, and then he would pay for my car home since he couldn't sleep with someone else in his bed. I didn't know if we were officially dating or not.

For lack of a better term, we were in a situationship.

And there's nothing I hated more than being in an ambiguous gray zone.

I invited him over a few days later to clarify things.

When he got to my apartment, there was a news report on in the background about a new #MeToo allegation.

"This stuff is crazy, ya know? Like, you can't do anything these days. The company I work for has stopped hiring women because we're so afraid of sexual harassment claims," he said.

I stared at him, dumbfounded.

"What do you mean?"

"You've got a bunch of programmers. They're awkward. They don't have, like, any experience with women. A girl joins the team and naturally they're flies to honey. They don't know they're sexually harassing someone."

My mouth dropped open.

"*Steve.* You're talking about adults. They know the difference between right and wrong. You can't just shrug your shoulders and be like, 'whoops, he didn't know that was inappropriate.'" I said, gritting my teeth. "And even if, *even if,* that was the case, shouldn't your solution be to educate them? Not a fucking ban on hiring women. Do you understand how this makes me feel? To know that women have fewer opportunities because some grown-ass men can't figure out how to not sexually harass someone?"

The argument escalated until I was too upset and could hardly speak. Steve wasn't listening; he was too focused on being right and making his point.

I stood up and glanced in the mirror. My face was covered in dark, blotchy hives, the kind I only got when I was feeling an intense emotion.

And then, despite myself, I began to rage cry.

I wanted to be a strong, bold woman who held her ground but I couldn't stop myself. I was *so mad*. The country was in crisis and what was playing out in the world was very much playing out in my own life. My argument with Steve was triggering the countless arguments I'd had on Facebook and in person. It was triggering the countless times I read comments where people made excuses about sexual assault and gender discrimination. I was tired of asking the same goddamned questions, again and again. Questions like: How could things change if we didn't start holding people accountable? How could young women believe they were smart and valuable, when both corporations and the justice system continued to fail them? How could I teach women that their voices and thoughts mattered when I couldn't even make a man I was intimate with listen to my voice or validate that my thoughts mattered?

In response, Steve stood up and hugged me tightly against his chest. It took everything I had not to punch him. I was mad at him but also mad at myself for crying. The only reason he was listening now was because I was feeding every stereotype about women being emotional and it was possibly invoking his need to protect me.

"It's frustrating. I know. It's gotta be frustrating," he said, stroking my back. He was trying to comfort me, but it felt condescending.

We sat down on the couch and he tried to soothe me, but I was still too mad. We turned on a sitcom to try to change the mood and sat there in silence for another thirty minutes barely talking to each other, before he pulled me closer to snuggle him. I didn't want to touch him. This issue was important to me and by not even trying to understand my perspective, I felt like he was part of the problem.

Despite my lack of reciprocity, he kissed me.

Before I knew it, he was dry humping me. He didn't give a shit or couldn't figure out that I didn't want that.

"Are you fucking kidding me?" I said, wiggling my way out from under him.

"Fucking really?" I said again, my hands on my waist, glaring at him.

"You need to leave," I said.

He tried to calm me down, but I wasn't budging. Then he had the audacity to say, "I want you to know how grateful I am to you for having these conversations with me. I want to be a better feminist. I want to advocate for women, so it's only through these conversations that I learn."

I wanted to slap him.

He left, and I was glad.

The next day Steve texted me again to apologize and tell me how "amazing, incredible, wonderful, and sexy" I was. It was the Steve lather, rinse, repeat cycle.

But I was done. If you can't defend my rights in public, you don't get to see my vagina in private.

I told him how upset I was about the night before and instead of empathizing, he doubled down on his point, trying to prove he was right. He said that I was being irrational and emotional, so of course, the whole argument was my fault. He followed that by thanking me for having hard conversations with him and helping him learn.

I was unimpressed by his emotionally manipulative bullshit, which I pointed out.

"I've never met someone who distrusted me as much you. I'm a good person. I don't need you to validate that," he said.

He was right. I distrusted him and did not think he was a good person.

I'd spent too much time and energy trying to make "this" work and even more energy trying to figure out what "this" was. I was still confused about all of it, everything from him cumming in his pants to the fact that he wouldn't stay over. Every time I thought about it, all I could think was, "What the fuck was that?"

He texted me a few more times, alternating between singing my praises and telling me how crazy I was before I blocked his number. Ain't nobody got time for that.

I was feeling too good about myself these days to put up with emotionally draining garbage.

Goodbye and good riddance.

I PAID A MAN TO
CUDDLE WITH ME

Affection was like Chinese food.

I could go long stretches without missing it at all, but once I had it again, I wanted to gorge myself. I had just eaten some Lo Mein of Love and now I wanted some Ecstasy Egg Rolls. Between Simon, Amit, and Steve, I'd seen more action the past year than the previous five years combined.

Of course, the cuddling experiment with Steve had turned into a cuddling calamity. Despite this, I wasn't quite done with cuddling yet.

Even though Steve was the worst, the few times we had platonically cuddled had done wonders. I couldn't forget those serene moments of oxytocin release.

In an attempt to fill my Chinese takeout carton of affection, I texted Amit. I hadn't seen him in almost two months. I'd been too involved with the Steve drama to follow up on his absenteeism.

He responded the next day with a text that was uncharacteristically short and evasive.

I turned into a Sherlock Holmes–CSI–Inspector Gadget and stalked his Instagram to see if I could get any hints about his disappearance. Had he been traveling for work? Kidnapped by Mafiosi? Working on a new EP for his cat?

The first picture was a fireplace with two pairs of slippers in front of it, one women's and one men's.

Ah, that's why I hadn't heard from him in a while. He had met someone.

"Hiii, are you still single?" I texted him, wanting confirmation.

"Oh fudge, I'm not," he wrote back immediately.

I was disappointed, but I couldn't be angry that he hadn't told me. I hadn't exactly told him about Steve.

"Oh wow, congrats!!" I texted back, sincerely.

"I loved exploring with you," he wrote a few minutes later.

"Likewise, wishing you nothing but the best," I typed back with a smiley face emoji.

It was an unceremonious ending, but what could I expect, a certificate of completion?

I guess all good Friends with Benefits must come to an end.

I was glad he had given me an opportunity to vulnerably discover sex. Our short-lived tryst had made me a more confident lover. While I was bummed about the loss of my FWB, I was ultimately happy for him. He was a good guy. He deserved someone who appreciated his cheesy puns.

Unfortunately, that meant I had no one to fool around or flirt with.

In a moment of desperation, I logged back into the Cuddling Cave.

My inbox was flooded again with men who wanted to pay me to cuddle.

Everyone offering to "buy my services" was over fifty or married, but it sparked the thought that maybe *I* could be the one to pay someone. I didn't want a repeat of Steve, where cuddling was a farce for hooking up, so if I really wanted uncomplicated, unemotional human touch—hiring someone seemed like a decent option.

I searched the site for professional male cuddlers and emailed the most popular one, Mike.

We scheduled an appointment, and two weeks later, I was in the middle of Queens on my way to meet him.

It was drizzling, and a depressing gray mist was covering the city. All the trees had lost their leaves and all the plants were dead. The garbage in the street was wet and stuck to the sidewalk. Spring was supposed to be here, but winter was hanging on fiercely to her reign.

As I walked the five blocks to his apartment, the reality of the situation set in: I was paying a man to cuddle with me.

In truth, I was hiring Mike 40 percent out of need for human touch and 60 percent out of Gemini curiosity. I wanted to meet a professional cuddler.

I double-checked the address on my phone and stopped in front of a well-kept building.

I buzzed his apartment. A feminine voice answered, "Hello?"

"Hi! I'm here for Mike."

"It's me! Come on up."

I climbed to the third floor, where I found Mike waiting for me at the top. He was tall and skinny with red streaks in his shoulder-length brown hair. He looked like the lead singer in a nineties alt-rock band. His place was boho chic with a brightly colored blue couch and macramé planters hanging in the kitchen.

His roommates were sitting in the living room playing video games. They ignored me, but I said hello anyway. No reason to make this awkward.

Despite the oddness of the situation, I wasn't embarrassed about hiring Mike. On the contrary, I thought it might save me from becoming *actually* desperate and winding up with another version of Steve.

The boho décor continued in his bedroom with purple and gold sheets. He had a salt lamp in the corner and the strong smell of sage hit my nose as we entered the room. There was a framed picture of him kissing a man in front of the Statue of Liberty.

He walked over to his computer and turned on some New Age music with rain sounds, turning up the volume just enough to cover the actual rain sounds.

"Today is all about you, honey," he said, reaching for a hug. "Do you have a side preference? Big spoon? Little spoon? Front, back?" he continued.

"I'd prefer to be on my stomach, please."

"Wonderful," he said, lying down on his back, fully clothed, on top of the covers. "You can join me whenever you're ready, honey."

I crawled in next to him and wrapped my arm over his chest.

He was sweaty and warm, but it still felt nice.

I was expecting it to be silent like it had been with Steve. Instead he asked me questions about my life, where I was from, my job. I answered and politely returned his inquiries.

I wanted to stop talking, but I couldn't figure out how to courteously say that. I spent ten minutes trying to figure out how to ask for silence before giving up and accepting the fact that we were going to chat the entire time. How classically Midwestern of me.

"How did you get into this?" I tried, figuring if we were going to talk, I might as well learn about professional cuddling.

"I wanted to help people. I believe that people are starved for affection and that causes a lot of problems for them. I get to be, like, a therapist and a healer, but with cuddling," he said rubbing my back.

Despite the physical closeness of our bodies, there was nothing sexual about the experience. We were holding each other. Nothing more, nothing less. I wondered if the talking was strategic, a way of ensuring that the experience remained professional and neutral.

He told me that he wasn't obligated to cuddle with anyone and he always screened his clients.

"What are most of your clients like?" I asked.

"Most are straight men," he said.

I raised my eyebrows, surprised by that answer. I expected his clients to be women in their thirties, like me, looking for extra affection.

"Straight men are the ones who are the most starved for human touch. Wanna move to spooning, honey?"

I rolled over, and as he arranged his body protectively around mine in "big spoon" formation, he told me that many of the men he cuddled with cried because they had never been held before.

"Wow, that's . . . heartbreaking," I said, letting out a sigh. I made a mental note to be the big spoon the next time I had someone to hold.

Ironically, while my little spoon position felt fine, I was missing the sexual tension. It was as platonic as it could possibly be, which was what I'd *thought* I wanted.

I turned and looked at his clock. We were ten minutes over our time. I knew he thought he was being generous, but my stomach was grumbling and there was a taco truck down the road calling my name.

"Oh, I think our sixty minutes are up. I don't want to monopolize your time," I said. It was one of the benefits of hiring someone; I didn't have to make up an excuse to leave.

"Thanks for pointing it out! Let's do the closing ritual."

Mike leapt off his bed and grabbed a large pink crystal. For the closing ritual we sat facing each other and held hands. We both had to say three things we were grateful for.

"I'm grateful for your ethereal being, the energetic magnitude of this moment, and the massive amount of love I feel pulsating through my body, today and always," Mike said, still clasping my hand.

"I'm grateful for you too, my family, and coffee. Amen," I said, with much less flair.

When I was done he held the pink crystal three inches away from my face and told me it would protect me from bad juju.

I thanked him with a hug, and we both got out of his bed and headed back down the hallway toward the front door.

His roommates were in the kitchen cooking a garlic stir-fry. They tried to ignore me as I walked by but I refused to be embarrassed, so I intentionally said, "Bye!" as I closed the door behind me.

As I was walking toward the taco truck, I received a text from Mike: "Had a great time!! Ten percent off for all repeat customers on their second visit!"

He was great but I didn't think there would be a second time, so I paid him on Venmo and thanked him for his services.

On the way home, I posted about my cuddling experience on Facebook. My friend Priya sent me a DM saying, "I'm interested in this platonic cuddling thing."

I recommended Mike, but when his fee was too high, she asked me if I knew anyone who might want to try it with her for free.

I had been chatting about it with one of my male friends a few days earlier, and he had also expressed fascination with the idea of platonic cuddling.

I connected them.

At my advice, they developed strict boundaries with timed sessions, open communication, and no staying over or kissing. They met twice a month and she contacted me a while later to say it had healed her from some deep trauma she had experienced earlier in her life.

I was happy to hear about her success; it was a reminder that it's possible to have two totally different experiences and not blame the experience itself. When it came to platonic cuddling, I'd had a terrible time with Steve; but Priya had amazing, life-altering encounters with her partner.

I thought about finding someone else to cuddle with but the more I thought about all of it, it occurred to me that I was trying to fool myself. What I truly wanted was a boyfriend. I wanted affection, love, and sex from one person who cared about me. I was trying, unsuccessfully, to fill in the gaps, and pretend that some half-starved form of tenderness was good enough.

It was time to start being honest with myself about what I really wanted.

TANTRA

I'd be honest with myself next week.

This week I had already scheduled my Tantra homework.

I grabbed my green research notebook, turned to a page in the middle, and wrote "Tantra Curriculum" in bold letters at the top.

When I was in high school, my best friend and I found a Kama Sutra book in her parents' bedroom. We studied the pages, not really understanding it, but believing that Tantra was the "next level" of sex.

Since I was trying to level up my lovemaking, Tantra had to be on the list.

The word *Tantra* itself means "expansion," "liberation," and "weaving." From what I could gauge, Tantra was the art of slow sex, created by "expanding one's own energy and weaving it with someone else's energy." Similar to OM'ing, it was about exploring pleasure without trying to arrive at a destination.

To get my feet wet, I went to an intro workshop where we partnered with a stranger and practiced gazing in each other's eyes. We spent a long time stroking each other's arms, and by the end, I did feel connected to my partner.

Afterward, I reached out to our instructor, Karen, for more information.

Karen agreed to meet me for coffee on a nondescript Tuesday at a nondescript Starbucks to continue discussing the benefits of slow sex.

Including her sexless marriage and subsequent divorce, Karen experienced a ten-year celibacy herself. She credited Tantra for helping her rediscover intimacy. She now believed that sexuality was a gateway to God.

At the end of our coffee date, I asked Karen for more resources, maybe a book, a YouTube video, or something.

"Tantra is more about mindset than anything else. There are many ways to explore but I'd recommend my favorite exercise: Find someone to stroke your naked body with a rose. For one full hour. No escalation, no reciprocity," Karen said nonchalantly, as if she'd just asked me to order her another coffee.

"Uh, I mean I would love to do that, believe me, I would *love* to do that. Alas, I'm currently very single so, um . . . is there like a book or something I could read?"

"I was single too the first time I did the rose ceremony. In fact, I did the ceremony with a total stranger I met that night. He was grateful for the opportunity," she said. "The point is for *you* to connect with your body and take without any obligation of having to give in return. That's what I'd recommend if you want to explore the tantra practice," she finished.

I tried to imagine the men I knew being grateful to participate in this corny Nicholas Sparks romance novel activity with me.

Yeah right.

Seeing the skepticism on my face, she said, "Put it out there; you might be surprised."

I doubted that was going to happen but nevertheless, I posted my homework on Facebook and asked if anyone was interested.

Within five minutes I received ten messages from friends and acquaintances offering to do the exercise with me.

"You know that I'm not going to return the favor in any sort of way, right? No kissing or anything," I sent to everyone who responded.

All the men still wanted to do the assignment.

I deliberated on the right person and finally settled on my friend Corwin. He was laid-back and easygoing. He was ten years older than me, though he could have passed for my age. He was young in spirit, loved loud concerts and staying out late. He was fit, handsome, and had a great sense of humor.

"I've always wanted to learn more about Tantra, I'd love to try this with you," he wrote.

Although we sometimes flirted, I didn't think Corwin was interested in dating or sleeping with me, which made it easier.

"We'll do the rose thing and then maybe get breakfast. But you understand that it isn't going to escalate past that?" I couldn't believe that anyone would want to do this thing with me, so I kept overexplaining it.

"You had me at breakfast," he wrote back. "My place or yours?"

I wanted to make it as convenient as possible for him, which meant his apartment.

On the night we were scheduled to meet, I took my time getting ready. I shaved my legs and carefully applied my makeup. It was the exact opposite of how I had treated the OM'ing exercise. This time, I wanted to feel attractive. In some ways, this exercise felt similar to OM'ing, at least the whole being present in your body thing. It was different because the purpose was to feel sexy and desirable, which wasn't a key component to OM'ing.

I looked at the list I had made in my notebook. It included some of the exercises we had discussed at the workshop and some things I had found online:

- Five minutes of joint breathing, fully clothed.
- Ten minutes of arm touching.
- Followed by him stroking me with the rose.

Karen hadn't recommended an agenda. She probably would have thought it was too clinical, but I couldn't help myself. I felt better with parameters; I guess old habits die hard.

I tore the paper out of my notebook and shoved it in my backpack before heading off to Corwin's. On the way, I stopped at my local bodega to buy a dozen pink roses.

I hopped on the train, flowers in hand, curriculum in bag, and headed toward Brooklyn.

"Beautiful flowers. Are they from your boyfriend?" an elderly woman sitting next to me asked.

I thought about telling her the truth but didn't want to scandalize her, so I just said, "Oh yes, he's wonderful."

"You're very lucky," she said.

She had no idea.

Corwin lived in a penthouse in a trendy area of Williamsburg. I arrived at a revolving set of doors that led to an expensive-looking lobby filled with plants. I went to text him that I was there but couldn't find my phone. I rifled through my bag and checked all my pockets three times. I dumped the entire contents of my backpack on the floor of his luxury apartment building, frantically flinging tampons, pens, and lip glosses across the entrance.

Not only was I addicted to my phone, but my phone case was also my wallet, which meant that I had no ID, no MetroCard, and no money.

Commence panic.

First and foremost, I was worried that someone was already using all of my credit cards to buy weird shit off Etsy and second, I was worried because it made me vulnerable.

Corwin and I were friendly acquaintances, but I didn't know him *that* well. What if things went off course and I needed to leave or call for help? What if I wound up in danger and had no way to escape? It occurred to me, for not the first time, that I had issues with safety.

I didn't know if it had to do with my paranoid parents or was just the by-product of being a woman, but I still felt unsafe around most men.

I didn't think Corwin was going to cross any boundaries or I wouldn't have been there, but even so, things could happen. I needed my phone. I sat down in the middle of his marbled lobby and clutched my bag to my chest. Without money or a MetroCard, I didn't have a lot of options.

I buzzed Corwin's apartment because there was nothing else I could do.

When he opened the door, before he could even hug me, I blurted out, "I lost my phone and my wallet and I'm freaking out."

"Oh shit, what do you want to do?" he said.

"Can I use your phone to cancel my cards?"

"Of course. Do you want to reschedule the rose thing for another night?"

"No, no. I'm already here, let's still do it."

He brewed some tea for me as I called my bank. After twenty minutes of screaming at automated messages, I tried to calm down for his sake because he seemed uncharacteristically nervous. We never had trouble chatting, but we were both being awkward and jumpy. I didn't know if he was picking up on my vibe, but this evening was off to a rocky start.

"Everything's good?" he asked.

"I think so. I can't do anything else about it tonight. Should we get started?"

We headed upstairs to his bedroom. Although I had been to Corwin's apartment many times, I had forgotten how incredible his room was. It was the size of my whole apartment with an entire wall of floor-to-ceiling windows and a private balcony that had a perfect view of the Manhattan skyline. He had art on his walls that he didn't buy at TJ Maxx. There was a sitting area with a classy couch and a bar. It was a gentle reminder that Corwin and I had very different-looking bank accounts. He never flaunted his wealth or made anyone feel bad about their own. In a city where people tried too hard to be impressive, that was something I really liked about him.

"What should I wear?" he asked.

"Whatever you want. Something comfortable," I said.

He changed into a light blue matching pajama set covered with cartoon owls. On anyone else it might have looked silly but on Corwin it looked good.

"Should we put on some music?" he asked, pacing the room.

Corwin was a music fanatic. I knew the right music would calm him down.

"Let me make a playlist." He kept checking in with me to make sure I approved of the song choices.

I sat on the edge of his California King, admiring the lights of the Empire State Building, trying not to worry about my missing phone and the fact that he was about to see me naked for the first time ever. We had never even kissed or touched each other a little too long. We were, at this point, purely friends, about to do this really intimate thing together.

When he finished his playlist, he joined me on the edge of the bed.

"So how does this work?" he asked.

"I've never done it before, so I'm not exactly sure, but I wrote out an agenda for us," I said, scrambling for my backpack to find the piece of paper I had shoved back in thirty minutes earlier.

"First we'll do some breathing exercises. We'll breathe in and out together and on the 'in' breath, we'll squeeze and hold our genitals."

I was repeating the instructions verbatim from a website about Tantra for beginners. I abbreviated the rest of the agenda, "Then some arm touching and finally the rose stuff. The whole thing will last sixty minutes, and everything is timed. Is that cool?"

"Of course," he said, smiling at me.

I looked at his face and saw, for possibly the first time, how kind his eyes were, how soft and gentle his face was. He had lines around his eyes and smile.

I looked at him looking at me and had a revelation. I had to stop treating this like he was doing me a favor. He wasn't; he wanted to be there. This was about owning my sexuality and taking without feeling guilty.

"Let's start with the breathing. Can you set a timer on your phone for ten minutes?"

We sat down facing each other in the middle of the bed, crisscross-applesauce style. I took his hands in mine and noticed how soft they were.

"Ready?" I asked.

He nodded.

I took a deep breath in sync with his and squeezed my pussy.* I could feel it tingle and wondered if Corwin's body was having a similar reaction. We breathed in and out, my breath mixing with his.

We repeated this, breathing in and exhaling together.

---

* At some point in time I transitioned from vagina to pussy since vagina wasn't technically the right terminology.

I wondered if breathing in sync meant that our hearts were beating in sync as well.

The timer went off and we both smiled at each other.

"Next is arm stroking, close your eyes and pay attention to the feeling of my hand on your arm," I said.

He stuck out his arm and I ran my fingers down it. I touched him intentionally, moving my hand softly down his arm toward his wrist before increasing the pressure. I tried to send all my energy out through my fingers and into his arm. When I arrived at his hand, I massaged his palm with my thumb before moving on to each individual finger.

Right when we were starting to connect and relax, the alarm buzzed. It dawned on me that maybe I was missing the point by using the alarm but I didn't know how to course correct and I was still too afraid that we'd get bored if we didn't use it.

"Your turn," Corwin said, interrupting my thoughts.

I stuck out my arm and closed my eyes as he massaged my arm.

His touch was light and gentle, but I couldn't focus.

I was worrying about my phone again. Someone was probably stealing my identity at that exact moment and getting free coffees with all of my customer loyalty cards.

I was ruining the whole thing by worrying.

If I had been alone, I probably would have let myself return to the rabbit hole of dread, but Corwin had agreed to do this with me and if I didn't calm down, I was wasting both his and my time.

I called on the focusing techniques I had learned during OM'ing (one of the most useful things I had learned) and put all my attention on the feeling of his fingers against my palm.

His index finger circled my wrist. Breathe.

His thumb rubbed my thumb. Breathe.

He massaged my hand. Breathe.

He stroked my pinky between two of his fingers, pulling it gently. Breathe.

The timer went off as I forgot all about my lost phone and wallet.

"Am I doing this right?" Corwin asked.

"You're doing it perfectly," I reassured.

I jumped off the bed and plucked one of the roses from the bouquet, handing it to Corwin.

"How should I stroke you? Like this?" Corwin asked holding the rose upright, "Or like this?" he said holding it at an angle.

"I think either one will be just fine," I said, smiling at his desire to do this properly. I liked that he was taking it seriously. He could have treated this like it was silly but he was making an effort, for both of us.

I peeled off my shirt and lay down in the middle of his bed in my best black pushup bra. I closed my eyes as I felt Corwin lower the rose to my collarbone. The rose petals felt cool and smooth on my skin. He ran the rose across my collarbone, over my bra, and down my stomach, repeating this pattern a few times. When the timer buzzed, I sat up, took in a deep breath and unhooked my bra, falling back into his smooth, Egyptian-cotton sheets. I thought I'd be nervous, but I wasn't. It felt luxurious to be partially naked in his extra-large bed, overlooking the Manhattan skyline.

Instead of nervous, I felt safe.

I was alone with him in his apartment, doing this crazy thing and I wasn't afraid. I wasn't worried that he was going to cross boundaries or make me feel disrespected. Corwin made me feel safe in a way I hadn't felt in a long time.

He slowly stroked the rose around the swell of my breast. Underneath it and then on top. He dragged the rose across my nipple, bringing it to a peak. It felt like silk being dragged across my body.

I arched slightly to meet the touch of the rose.

Seeing my response, he replicated the same pattern for the next ten minutes, running the rose over the swell of my breast, pausing slightly at my nipples. I relaxed into the sensation, appreciating the repetition.

The alarm buzzed, signaling that it was time to remove the rest of my clothes.

While I was definitely savoring the sensations, I wasn't feeling overtly aroused. Perhaps I had made the whole thing too platonic by adding in the timer and reiterating, ad nauseam, that it wasn't going to escalate.

"I'm going to get fully naked now, okay?" I said checking-in with Corwin.

"Yep."

I peeled off my pants and my underwear and lay back down.

I closed my eyes as Corwin dragged the rose down my stomach, stopping above my thigh.

He hesitated, seemingly uncertain where he should stroke.

I opened my legs slightly to let him know it was okay and he carefully touched the rose to my inner thigh.

He stopped again, for only a second, before rubbing it slowly around my outer labia. He went back to my thigh before circling back again. He continued this for several minutes and finally my body responded with heat. A small moan escaped my lips as he circled my thigh one final time before the alarm buzzed.

That was the end of the sixty minutes.

I lay there for a second before rolling over. Even though I was undressed, I didn't feel vulnerable so I motioned for him to lay down next to me. When he did, I scooched my body close to his and rested my head on his pajama-clad chest.

"Thank you," I said, looking him in the eyes.

"My pleasure," he replied.

A wave of tiredness hit me as I looked at the clock. It was 1:30 a.m. I snuggled closer, burying my face against him.

"Your chest feels like clouds," I said drowsily, yawning into his body.

He wrapped me in his arms and we both fell asleep, nestled together. Me fully naked, him fully clothed.

I woke up a few hours later and accidentally woke Corwin in the process. I sat up, stretched, and said, "I should get going."

It was late and I was tired, but I knew I shouldn't stay and he didn't invite me to.

Forever the gentleman, he offered to pay for a car home since I didn't have my wallet.

He walked me to the door and hugged me goodbye.

I fell asleep on the way home and realized my dreams were about roses and Corwin's cloud-like chest. I wasn't fantasizing about him or wishing he'd ask me out but I was grateful. Losing my phone, in some ways, meant losing control. As a recovering control freak, that was hard for me. I had to trust Corwin. And he lived up to it by not pressuring me and making me feel safe. The whole point of the Tantra exercise was about letting someone care for me and feeling beautiful in the process. Corwin had created a space that felt secure enough for me to relax and feel sexy.

I woke up late the next morning and when I checked my Facebook, I had a message from someone who had found my phone. They returned it, all of the cards fully intact.

I texted Corwin, who wrote, "See, people can be good. You gotta trust, Olive."

Compared to where I'd started, I was feeling pretty good about my progress.

SQUIRTING LAB

The liquid that comes from a woman while squirting both is and is not pee.

At least that's what I wrote down during the first part of the Squirting Playlab. I was the only one taking notes and only one of four people who wasn't part of a couple.

The Squirting Playlab was precisely what it sounded like. The promise was to teach participants how to make their partner squirt, assuming their body was capable of that sort of thing, which apparently, with the right moves, many bodies were.*

Only in NYC could someone's Friday night involve dollar pizza and a squirting class.

Going to the Squirting Playlab was simultaneously the best and worst idea I'd ever had. It was a great idea because I was interested in squirting. It was a terrible idea because it involved learning to squirt in a room full of other people.

Also, in this class, it was a two-person activity and I was unattached.

I had been on two dates with a boy recently, but I could hardly ask him.

---

* It's also possible to make yourself squirt, but this was a partner-focused class.

I imagined how that conversation might go, "Hey, I know this is only our third date but wanna go to a squirting class with me? Oh yeah, I forgot to tell you, I'm writing a book about crazy sex stuff, so, see you at nine and bring goggles."

No thanks.

I'd have to fly solo and cross my fingers that maybe some dreamboat was also at the class, flying solo. Maybe we'd fall in love and then we'd have to make up a totally different "how we met" story to tell our grandchildren.

A girl could dream.

Up until that point, almost everything I had done, I had done privately, excluding the BDSM class, which felt light years away. In reality, it had been about a year and a half. It was one thing to learn and then try out the skills behind closed doors. It was a totally different thing to ejaculate maybe/maybe-not pee in a room full of people. Doing something this bold in public made me feel like I was finally ready to leave the sex kiddie pool. Either that or I'd been on this voyage for too long and I'd lost my damn mind. Either way I was diving in.

The Playlab was held at La Casa, a prominent player in the New York sex-positive scene. Renee was a member and spoke highly of the community. La Casa hosted workshops, seminars on ethical non-monogamy, and sex parties. It was also a residential community for people who wanted to live with other sex-positive people.

La Casa was located in a discreet apartment building in the East Village. I arrived fifteen minutes before class and paced outside before entering. Despite my false bravado, I was a beginner compared to these people. I was worried that everyone else was going to be La Casa regulars, people who attended orgies and had long ago made peace with their sexuality.

Maybe I should have stayed in the kiddie pool.

La Casa had no identifying markers of being a sex-positive community. On the outside it looked like a regular apartment building. I rang the doorbell and was invited inside and asked to remove my shoes.

I walked down a flight of stairs into a large room filled with oversized, purple velvet cushions. There was a chandelier in the middle of the room and fancy curtains covering the windows. There was an outdoor patio with a hot tub, a luxury I had *never* seen at a residential property in New York City. It seemed like no expense had been spared in turning La Casa into a swanky sex haven.

There were some couples seated on the cushions, talking quietly among themselves and kissing occasionally.

There was an uncomfortable silence over the room. It was clear we were all uncertain how to behave. I must have been wrong about the class being full of sex-positive regulars.

I thought about being the badass who broke the ice, but instead I did what everyone else was doing and took forever to set down my stuff, went to the bathroom a few times, and hovered near the food table.

When I'd finally run through all my avoidant behaviors, I plopped myself down next to the only other solo person there and introduced myself.

His name was Willie. He looked older than me with gray hair and wrinkle lines on his forehead. Like me, Willie was tired of being alone and scared of sex.

I had met many people like Willie, comrades in sexual experimentation, celibates, and inexperienced amateurs. We'd run into each other in the different scenes, in person at workshops or online, registered on Fetlife. Most of us had fallen into this world accidentally, desperate to save ourselves. Some of us had become good friends. We often compared notes and lamented about how much easier this would be if we were in relationships. Two more unaccompanied men filtered in. So far, I was the only single woman. In addition to us solo players, there were about ten couples, eager and ready to learn.

Willie left to grab food, and within two minutes, one of the other single men sat down next to me. Unlike Willie, he was sitting a little too close.

As I was trying to avoid the new guy's advances, a couple walked in. I recognized the woman but couldn't figure out how. I was racking my brain, running through the sexy adventures I'd had in the last few months, trying to place her.

It took a few seconds, but I realized that she was an HR director at one of my biggest corporate clients. I had taught her and her team public speaking in a very professional way. I didn't recognize her because she was out of context here.

My palms started getting sweaty and I could feel the blush spreading up my face.

I'd only ever seen this woman in a suit and she'd only ever seen me buttoned-up as well.

Here we were, at a squirting class together.

I felt like I'd been caught in the act. I wondered if I was going to have to tell my boss.

As I deliberated about how to handle the situation, she walked up and gave me a big hug.

"Olive, it's so wonderful to see you!" she said.

She introduced me to her husband. We chatted about public speaking and how she'd used the tips I'd given her. She was cheerful and unapologetic, so I followed her lead.

We chatted a little more before our instructor, Thomas Lovefell, entered the room, his long hair tied up in a ponytail. I doubted that was his real name as it was pretty common in the sex-positive world to have an alias. Thomas was famous in the sex-education world, handsome yet accessible. I'd seen him shirtless on the Internet, and the man was ripped.

The class was divided into three parts: lecture, live demo, and practice playtime.

The lecture was a PowerPoint. It defined squirting, reviewed techniques, and included time for Q&A. Nerd that I was, I took copious notes, Harriet the Spy style.

Despite listening to a lecture for half an hour about the topic, I still couldn't figure out if it was pee. From what I could determine, the fluid that came out of a woman while squirting came from the bladder but wasn't exactly urine. It was secreted from some gland that I couldn't remember the name of and a woman could empty her bladder and still squirt. It wasn't similar to urine in smell or color. Despite this, no one had specifically said, "No. It isn't pee."

After the PowerPoint portion ended, Thomas was going to demonstrate the squirting techniques on his partner Luly.

Without saying anything, just by the way she had walked into the room—shoulders back, head up—it was clear that she was fierce. She looked like someone who would have worked at the Dominatrix Den. She was a buxom babe with wild, curly hair that framed her face and demanded attention, kind of like Luly herself. She was wearing a corset on top and lacy underwear on the bottom; nothing like the granny panties I was wearing.

Thomas rolled out a white massage table covered in disposable, absorbent pads, like the kind used to train puppies. The whole setup looked sterile and uncomfortable. Given the luxe design of La Casa, I was expecting it to be sexier.

The puppy pads were throwing me off. I imagined a couple in the bedroom, passionately making love, when one of them stopped to grab the puppy pads.

Sex was messy, and I liked that. In my own life, I think I'd prefer to soak the sheets, but I could appreciate how clean and sterile La Casa was. Despite frequent sex parties, it was probably more sanitary than my own apartment.

Luly took off her clothes, climbed on the table, and lay down.

The class crowded around the massage table, Luly naked and resting in the middle. She didn't feign modesty or pleasure.

Thomas instructed everyone to start touching their partners, to become familiar with their bodies and genitals. He wanted to heighten the sexual energy in the room.

As the couples started massaging and groping each other, I stood there with my hands folded across my chest.

Noticing me, Thomas said, "If you're alone, touch yourself."

I wasn't sure where to look so I closed my eyes and slid my hand down my leg. I wanted to enjoy it, but I was feeling self-conscious about my single status.

Apparently, I wasn't the only one. The second single man I had chatted with came over and whispered in my ear, a little too loudly, asking if I wanted to be his partner.

I didn't. It seemed weirder to fake intimacy than just accept that I was alone.

I said, "No thanks." Still, he hovered for several minutes as I continued to ignore him.

"Squirting isn't necessarily an orgasm," Thomas explained, touching Luly's thighs.

"Both feel pleasurable, but not necessarily the same," Luly chimed in, her voice crisp and clear.

That was news to me. I'd always assumed that squirting was a powerful orgasm, like the top tier of orgasms. He was going to make her squirt first and then make her squirt and orgasm at the same time to demonstrate the differences.

He started stimulating her, inserting his fingers into her pussy in the proper position, hitting her G-spot. She didn't seem too aroused; in fact, she looked a little bored.

"I'm going to externally stimulate Luly a little more," he said, rubbing her clitoris and nipples.

Her face flushed as she started showing more visible signs of arousal.

"Now I'm going to head back in internally and make her squirt," he said as he placed his fingers back in her pussy. Sure enough, a few moments later a spray of fluid gushed from her vagina onto the puppy pads. The fluid was white and milky, and, as promised, didn't smell or look like urine.

As spectators, we weren't sure what to do. It felt like the time I had accidentally watched *American Pie* with my parents: I didn't want to move or breathe the wrong way. I looked down at the floor and pretended to pick some lint off my top.

"Let's give Luly a round of applause!" Thomas said.

We applauded politely, as Thomas removed the puppy pad and replaced it with another one.

"Do you need a second or should we continue the demo?" he asked, turning toward Luly.

"Continue the demo," Luly said, wiping sweat from her brow.

Thomas grabbed a large instrument from the bottom of the massage table. It was a Hitachi Magic Wand, and I knew that meant things were about to get serious.

"Now let me show you squirting *with* an orgasm," he said.

He positioned the vibrator against her clitoris, rubbing her thighs and getting her ready for round two. He rotated between stimulating her internally and rubbing her clit.

This time around she seemed anything but bored. Her face contorted, and she started moaning and screaming. We were instructed to move outside of the "splash zone." It took only a few minutes before she sprayed the entire table with fluid. The puppy pads were soaked and some liquid splashed onto the floor.

It was the first time I had ever seen another female orgasm live. I had watched plenty of porn but watching Luly was a totally different experience. It was both arousing and intimate.

This time we all clapped without being prompted. It seemed odd but it would have been even weirder to just stand there and not acknowledge anything.

We took a break so Luly could clean up. The next part was for couple's only. They were going to practice the techniques. I desperately wanted to stay but wasn't allowed because I was partner-less. This was technically a couple's class so they were trying to protect against voyeurs.

I had made an agreement with myself at the beginning of the Coitus Chronicles that it wasn't going to be scholarly. This had to be experiential; otherwise it was all phony. Sitting on the sidelines taking notes without trying things was disrespectful. If I did that, I was Busybody Bettie, someone who could easily extract herself from any stigmas by using the excuse "I'm here because I'm writing a book."

No. I wasn't going to do that. I needed to come back to class, this time with a partner.

I returned to the Playlab a few months later with Corwin. I had seen him only once since the Tantra exercise, at a cookout where I told him about the Playlab. He was always curious about sexual things, so he offered to go with me. He had already seen me naked, so it didn't seem like too big of a leap to make.

He joined me at La Casa for the next class.

We watched the lecture and demo together.

After they asked all the single people to leave, I was over the moon that I got to stay this time. It felt like I was a member of a secret club of evolved, next-level sex-ers.

I high-fived Corwin.

"Go ahead and start to undress," Thomas instructed.

Corwin had already seen me in my birthday suit but no one else in the room had. I did my best to not feel self-conscious and laid down on a puppy pad.

My stomach started growling, even though I had eaten before class.

I heard Thomas giving instructions but I couldn't listen; my heart was beating too loudly in my head. Corwin was clasping his hands and trying to look cool but I could feel his nervous energy as well.

I couldn't relax. I still wasn't comfortable with public displays of sexuality. Not to mention, Corwin and I weren't lovers. The more I thought about it, it was an astronomical, Grand Canyon–sized leap to go from a privately shared Tantra exercise to learning to squirt in public. I wasn't ready, might never be ready, to be in a room where other people could see me maybe/maybe-not pee all over a puppy pad.

I sat up abruptly, the blood rushing to my face, and whispered to Corwin, "I don't think I can do this."

"Yeah, it's a little much, huh?" he whispered back.

I didn't want to make it awkward by leaving but if there was one lesson I had truly gotten from all my explorations, it was that you never had to do things you didn't want to do.

"Let's leave."

"Of course," he said.

We got up and I quickly dressed, thanked Thomas for the class, and told him we were going to try the technique at home. Whether I wanted to be or not, I was still a lady-in-the-streets, freak-in-the-sheets kind of gal.

"Wanna go get ice cream?" I asked, turning to Corwin.

"Hell yes, that's the best idea we've had all day."

"Agreed," I said, dragging him by the hand toward the ice cream store around the corner.

I wasn't fully done with squirting. I resolved to try it.

At home.

Behind closed doors.

Without puppy pads.

With my next boyfriend. If there ever was one.

EVERYONE TOLD ME NOT TO DO IT AND I DID IT ANYWAY

E xes are a bad idea.

I knew this.

I told all my friends this when they hooked up with their exes.

And yet . . .

I hadn't seen or talked to Simon in eight-or-so months when we decided to try the friend thing. He commented on one of my Facebook statuses which resulted in me sliding into his DMs and now we were meeting up as *just friends.*

After all, couldn't two adults who enjoyed each other's company be friends?

We met for dinner and coffee at a Whole Foods. Nothing could be more platonic than eating under fluorescent lights with a bunch of screaming toddlers.

On the day of, I arrived fifteen minutes early and paced a block away before finally heading toward our meeting spot.

I saw him standing by the flowers, looking handsome in a tan button-down shirt. My stomach clenched and the pit of nerves in my belly turned into a sick feeling.

You can do this, I thought walking through the front doors. *You're just going to act like you would with any other friend.*

I walked up and gave him a cautious hug.

"Hey! So good to see you," I said too enthusiastically.

"You too!" he said, matching the fakeness in my own tone.

We both ordered medium coffees, grabbed dinner from the buffet, and sat on a bench, side-by-side, as we had done many times before. Luckily, the smell of BBQ tofu wafting from the next table over killed any romantic ambiance.

"So, how's your job and stuff?" I asked.

"Good, good, got a real nine-to-five now and everything. How's yours?"

He seemed as nervous as I was: we were both talking too fast and trying too hard to act normal.

After we had covered all the basics, he asked, "How's the book coming along?"

I avoided looking at him, pushing my rice around the to-go container with my fork.

What he meant was, "Have you written a chapter about me yet?" He knew it was inevitable after being the one to break the dry spell.

"Oh yeah, good, good . . ." was all I could manage to say.

He looked me squarely in the face and said, "Listen, I knew there was a chance you were going to write about me. I was in a bad place and I was a jackass. So, write the story how you need to. You don't have to protect me."

I scanned his eyes, assessing the sincerity of his statement. I was moved by the gesture. The sick feeling in my stomach went away, replaced by gratitude.

"We both know I'm going to," I said.

His face softened in response.

"You gotta stop trying to protect everyone. And for the love of God, stop thinking so damn much, my dear."

I laughed. We were infamous for our overthinking. It was probably the death of all of our relationships.

After that, we both relaxed and caught up on all the crazy stuff that had happened in the past several months, though I carefully left out my dating life.

Coffee turned into dessert and dessert turned into a walk. Conversation was easy, like it had always been. I was glad we were hanging out; I had missed him.

"That was fun," he texted me after I left.

"Agreed, let's do it again sometime."

Sometime came a month later and then again a few weeks after that. We weren't contacting each other regularly, but we weren't avoiding each other as vigilantly as we had been. It was sporadic. Random drinks. Coffee in the park.

It was all friendly until one night we got drunk on sake and someone grabbed someone's hand.

Someone kissed someone.

Before I knew it, we were doing the Cupid Shuffle all over again. To the right, to the right, *to the right back to where we left off.*

A few weeks later we went to the museum to celebrate his birthday.

I was déjà vu-ing in front of the Picassos to the date we'd had almost a year ago.

We sat down on a bench, and he brushed his lips across mine. I ran my fingers over the scar on this face.

We spent three hours meandering around the museum, debating the merits of Rauschenberg and admiring the Van Goghs before deciding to get dinner.

After eating, we stood on the sidewalk, sheltered from the rain, and kissed in a way we hadn't kissed each other in a long time. It was deep, sensual, and caring. Our bodies were responding with heat and desire.

As his tongue grazed mine, I slid my hand up his back, underneath his shirt, rubbing his skin with need and desire.

He leaned over and kissed my neck. "God, I want to be inside of you," he whispered.

Less than five minutes later, we were in a cab back to his apartment. He pulled off my shirt the minute we walked in the door. We were both fully naked before we had even hit his bedroom, clothes strewn all over his apartment for his roommate to find.

Our bodies rocked in sync until we both came.

Afterward, he reached for me and I went to him, soaking in the warmth of his body.

As we lay there, talking and holding each other, I could feel my heart beating a little too fast.

I was playing with fire. We still hadn't clarified what we were doing. We didn't contact each other every day. We didn't see each other every week. I had no idea if he was dating other people. I wasn't even sure if we were dating.

A week later he invited me over for dinner. He met me at the train station and walked me to his house where I was greeted with the smell of roasted chicken and potatoes. He'd spent all day getting ingredients from various farmers' markets. Fresh rosemary and basil. Artisan chocolate and whiskey for dessert. Because I was looking for clues about what he and I were, it seemed like a good sign.

We cooked together, both of us taking turns reading the recipe and seasoning the potatoes.

When dinner was done cooking, we sat down on the couch, ready to eat.

"How's your love life? Any new prospects?" he asked, casually, scooping some potatoes on to his fork.

I raised by eyebrows in confusion; talk about sending mixed signals.

"It's fine. How's yours?" I said in a tone that attempted to convey that this wasn't something I wanted to talk about.

"Well, there was this one friend of mine, Angie. We tried to hook up and it was a disaster. It was sitcom-level awkward," he said, laughing, making it clear that he was telling me because he thought I'd appreciate the joke of how catastrophic it had all been.

Maybe I was being an ol' stick in the mud, but I didn't see the humor.

He pulled out his phone, "It was such a wreck that it warranted an email to my dad," he said, passing it to me so I could read the "hilarity."

Goddamnit, Simon.

I stood up, grabbed my plate, and headed toward the kitchen to start cleaning the pots and pans. With my back to him, I placed my plate in the dishwasher. I was silent for a long time before I said, "I don't really want to read that. And I definitely, definitely don't want to know about girls you fucked, or tried to fuck, or are trying to fuck."

"I think you're overreacting. I mean, I wouldn't be upset if you told me about one of your lovers," he replied.

What the fuck, man.

"Well, you and I are different," I said.

"Okay, of course. I just thought, you know, because we're friends, we could talk about this stuff. Like, I told all my other friends about the debacle with Angie."

So, we were doing this. Pretending like we had zero history and we were just two people who hooked up when we were drunk.

When I didn't say anything, he filled the silence by digging a deeper hole.

"Olive, I love your company. I get hard thinking about you. But one of the biggest problems I have with our friendship is that I can't talk to you honestly about myself without hurting your feelings," he replied.

One of my biggest problems was that we were sleeping together, and he was still referring to it as a friendship.

"We don't make sense in a relationship," I said to save face, despite the fact that earlier that morning I was considering the possibility of getting back together. "But we aren't friends; we're exes. And goddamnit, Simon, I'm a person and I have an ego. Do you understand how confusing this all is for me?" I said making a sweeping gesture toward the chocolate and the rest of the meal on the stove.

He looked around as if he'd just realized how I'd interpret this whole night.

I sighed heavily.

Right then and there I made a choice. I wasn't doing this.

Old me might have put up with this crap and rationalized, *Well, technically we aren't in a relationship, and I didn't ask him for clarity, so I don't have any right to be mad.*

But I was mad. I wasn't going to stand there and pretend like we were hookup buddies and that having sex with him wasn't meaningful for me. I wasn't going to let him invalidate my feelings so that he could say and do whatever he wanted.

I had to be honest with myself that Simon was never going to be who I needed and we were both wasting our time in a way that was only hurting me.

"Thank you for the meal," I said, grabbing my coat and heading for the door.

I was proud of myself for having the courage to leave. I'm not sure that's something I would have done two years ago.

Later that night when I was in bed, I was still mad at Simon, but mostly I was mad at myself.

I was repeating the same patterns of behavior. As a result, I kept winding up in one-sided, confusing situations with emotionally unavailable lovers who could take me or leave me.

I gave and they took.

I called it casual when, for me, it wasn't.

I worried.

I cried.

I analyzed.

But I didn't change.

It was like watching the same movie, over and over but with different characters.

I thought of all the men before and after Simon. Amit, Ben, Steve. I was grateful for how they helped me rediscover intimacy and realize what I wanted and didn't want from a partner. They were all valuable learning experiences.

Now, I had to demand better.

I had to raise the standards on my love life. I knew that if I didn't, I was never going to find a partner.

This wasn't just about sex anymore. It was about finding someone I could have a healthy, loving, sexually intimate relationship with.

This was the turning point.

I was ready to find love.

AN ENDING THAT'S HAPPY

spent a long time thinking about how I wanted this book to end. I wanted this to be a story of self-discovery, with glimmers of sadness and sparkles of hope. Just enough sexiness to make it spicy. And of course, a little bit of humor.

When I wrote the original ending, it was an anthem for single people. I was happy and optimistic. I believed that someone was out there for me and when the universe was good and ready, I'd find the Amal to my Clooney. The Jim to my Pam. But at the time that I wrote it, there wasn't anyone. There was no starry-eyed story arc or knight in shining armor. My life was good and that was enough.

Then, six months before this book was due, I met Jamie.

He had wavy hair and warm, dark eyes. He was a sexy nerd who was obsessed with sport fencing and could solve a Rubik's Cube in under a minute.

We met through OkCupid and while I wasn't swooning on our first date, it was good enough for a second date. As time passed it was clear that he was remarkably kind, thoughtful, funny, and loving. Our second date rolled into a third date and before I knew it, he was calling me his girlfriend.

No one had *ever* introduced me as their girlfriend.

He made it easy to be with him. He texted me every day, unlike Simon. He never crossed boundaries like Steve. He wanted to explore, like Amit. I never once felt insecure or uncertain about whether he wanted to be with me. I wore a baseball cap on our first date and he told me how beautiful I looked and made me feel beautiful subsequently every day after that.

One day when I was lost, and Google Maps wouldn't work on my phone, I called Jamie. He looked up my destination online and gave me directions for thirty minutes, calling himself my personal GPS and staying on the phone until I arrived at where I was going.

He'd sneak chocolate bars into my bag, he'd tell me how proud he was of me, and he bought me a phone charger for his place. He was always doing thoughtful things like that for me.

He showed up in ways no one ever had. After two months of dating, my roommates and I were moving apartments again. As Jamie carried down my eleventh box from my fourth-floor walk-up, in the pouring rain, he never once complained. When he was done moving my stuff, he headed back upstairs to grab Lindsay and Mary's boxes as well. I kissed him on the front stairs, rain dripping off his nose, and said, "I'm the luckiest." At my new apartment, he built my bed and hung my shelves.

The first time we had sex he attended to me with great care and finesse. It was electrifying and loving. He stroked my face and held me until the morning.

In some ways, Jamie felt like my final exam at the end of the semester.

After two years of sex research, both academic and experiential, I was able to try out my newfound skills. Everything I had learned in classes and every position I had failed with other people. I was finally comfortable and vulnerable and because of that, we were having the best sex of my life.

He wanted to explore with me, so we tried everything:

Girl on top, couldn't stop.

We used pineapples and mango skins.

We did it in the shower.

Every hour.

In the kitchen.

On the floor.

Foot stuff.

Behind the door.

We tried it all. We'd effortlessly move from doggy to missionary to some crazy move I'd never done before and couldn't name. He made me cum six times in one night, went to sensation play classes with me, and watched videos on OM'ing.

On a chilly fall weekend, I rolled over and snuggled against his chest, "Okay, this is weird, but I have a thing about reverse cowgirl."

"What do you mean?" he asked twisting a piece of my hair around his finger.

"I don't know, I'm worried that everyone knows how to do it but me."

"Maybe we should practice until you feel confident?" he asked, rolling me over and kissing my neck. We did it four or five times that week until I felt like I had mastered the position.

He said he loved me after three months. When I told him I wasn't there yet—that it felt too soon, that I was someone who took things slow—without guilting me or acting hurt, he said, "You don't have to say it back, baby. There's no rush. I want you to always be honest with how you feel about me, and I'll always be honest with you."

It was a perfect response; instead of bolting like I'd normally do, it made me fall for him even more.

On Valentine's Day he gave me a custom-made stamp with my initials on it and ordered a Brazilian pastry that I had mentioned I missed, once, in passing, several months before. Jamie remembered things like that. After I opened the bag, I smiled and said, "I think I love you too," and I meant it.

It's still new, so I won't pretend this is a set-in-stone fairy-tale ending, but I'm happy. After two years of searching, failing, exploring, confronting old beliefs, changing, and growing, I found someone who loves me and who I love back.

And just like that, easier than it all began. . . .

My Coitus Chronicles had come to an end.

ACKNOWLEDGMENTS

It's 11:52 pm, three months before this book is coming out, and I've been putting off writing this all day. Instead I cleaned my apartment, called my friend, reorganized that one drawer. My procrastination comes from the fact that this is possibly the most important thing I'll write in this whole book.

When I think about what I'm most grateful for it's always: 1. My relationships and 2. The ability to make art, to use my words to create things that help people or make them laugh. In some way, this is a combination of both of those things.

So, how do I express how deeply fucking grateful I am to all these people who have given me the gift of their talent, friendship, and love? It's much easier to organize that drawer.

Like anything in writing, to start, you just start. So here it goes:

To my mom, I'm so lucky to be your daughter, not only did you teach me how to be a funny storyteller, you taught me how to be independent and smart. Love you always, more than you can imagine. To dad, you taught me to dream big, and that belief and support is THE direct cause of this book. From one artist to another, proud to be an Alexander. Ian, my other dad, you're the rock. Thanks for always slipping me twenties and not getting angry about that time I drove across the lawn accidentally. Leah, you're funnier than I am, I love that we're getting closer as we get older, may that only continue. To the rest of my family: God, I love us. Seriously, other people's families are so fucked up, but we're pretty functional. Also, thanks for being cool that I write about sex. That's really freaking hard, but you all have only ever supported me in the "We're your biggest cheerleaders EVER" sort of way.

To my agent, Myrsini, at Carol Mann, thank you believing in this book, and me, before it was even a thing. It means more than I know how to say.

To my editor, Caroline, and the entire team at Skyhorse, thanks for all the time, energy and love put into this book. Thank you for always accepting my meetings in-person.

To Jason and the entire team at Brilliance, holy shit, there's going to be an audio version of this book. OMFG, that's the most exciting thing ever.

Kymian, Katharine, Liz, Nikki, Nathan, thank you for reading countless chapters and offering your HONEST feedback. It was invaluable, as is your friendship. Vern, you get your own line. Thanks for your unconditional kindness, even when I was grumpy. Marina, thanks for being a great coach and always getting my ass into gear.

To all my friends in Ohio, you know who you are, thank you for making it feel like I never left every time I come home. It's one of the main reasons I'm able to still use the word HOME. You're stuck with me forever. Can't wait to be ninety-five and sitting around Tony's basement the night before Thanksgiving.

To all my friends in NYC, you know who you are, thank you for making this a place that also feels like home. To the countless times you showed up to parties. The countless times you answered your phones and came to my shows. To my communities, from PDN to HTM, thank you for providing consistent friendship and support all these years.

To all my friends elsewhere, Hi, I miss you. I love you. Call me soon?

To all the men who cared about me, thank you for teaching me both what healthy and unhealthy relationships look like. For helping me see what you saw. To JMM, thank you for teaching me what it looked like to both love and show up for another person.

To God, for my health, the good health of the people I love, and well, everything. To Millie, George, Grandma G, Webster, Paula, Phyllis, Faigy, Lisa, John, Margaret and all the other angels, thank you for always listening to my prayers. Catch you in the next life when we're all cats.

To everyone on the internet who supported not only my work, but this whole journey, thank you. From the bottom of my heart, thank you. I read every comment, laugh at your wittiness, and feel like I've developed honest Facebook friendships with many of you.

Finally, to everyone who wants to write a book: Do it. It doesn't matter if you have a platform or not. It doesn't matter if anyone has validated whether or not you should. It doesn't matter how flushed out your idea is or if you suck at grammar. Do it anyway and figure it out as you go. Write because that's what you were put on this earth to do.

With every ounce of my being, Thank you all.